AN ANNOTATED BIBLIOGRAPHY OF DANCE/MOVEMENT THERAPY:

1940 - 1990

by

Heidi Fledderjohn, M.A., DTR, and Judith Sewickley, M.A., DTR

Marian Chace Memorial Fund

of the

American Dance Therapy Association

Columbia, Maryland

REF. 615.85155 F593a c. 2

Fledderjohn, Heidi.

An annotated bibliography of dance/movement therapy,

Copyright © 1993

by

Heidi Fledderjohn, Judith Sewickley,

and the
Marian Chace Memorial Fund of the
American Dance Therapy Association
2000 Century Plaza
Columbia, Maryland 21044

All rights reserved.

Cover graphics: Franklin Londin
John Roll

Library of Congress Catalog Card Number:
93-080089

ISBN: 1-881766-03-9

CONTENTS

ACKNOWLEDGEMENTS..i
INTRODUCTION..ii

<u>Section</u>   <u>Page</u>

A. THEORETICAL AND RESEARCH MATERIAL
    IN DANCE/MOVEMENT THERAPY..................................1

        Conference Proceedings and Monographs................38

B. CLINICAL PRACTICE
    IN DANCE/MOVEMENT THERAPY.................................43

<u>Chapter</u>   <u>Page</u>

    1. Adolescent Disorders..........................43
    2. Anxiety Disorders.............................46
    3. Childhood Disorders...........................47
    4. Eating Disorders..............................59
    5. Family..61
    6. Geriatrics....................................63
    7. Mood Disorders................................68
    8. Neuroses......................................69
    9. Personality Disorders.........................73
    10. Physical and Sexual Abuse.....................75
    11. Schizophrenia.................................76
    12. Somatic Disorders.............................85
    13. Substance Abuse...............................87
    14. Traumatic Brain Injury........................89

Appendix A..90

ACKNOWLEDGMENTS

The authors wish to acknowledge the following people who were crucial to the development of this project: Anne Fisher, for applying her research knowledge in dance/movement therapy, and Arnie Sanders, for helping the authors recognize and remember the value of the work. Appreciation is also extended to the Marian Chace Memorial Fund for publishing this project.

The following people graciously shared important information from their respective fields: Dr. Katie Killeen, whose expertise in child psychology aided in creating an accurate research tool, Dr. Richard Pringle, for his understanding of the American Psychological Association bibliographic format, and Marjorie Simon at the Goucher College Library for assisting in the beginning stages of the project.

The authors are sincerely grateful to their families for their support and encouragement: Joan Sewickley and Thomas DiBernardi, and Don, Linda, Gretchen and Erica Fledderjohn. Finally, the authors wish to express special thanks for the kindness, caring, and ongoing support of Kirk Mangels and Jerome Bolkcom.

INTRODUCTION

The intent of this annotated bibliography is to present published literature that includes clinical, theoretical and research material in the field of dance/movement therapy. It is intended for clinicians and students in the field, as well as other mental health professionals interested in the clinical, theoretical and research aspects of dance/movement therapy. The scope of the literature spans the years 1940 to 1990.

The authors chose the years 1940 to 1990 as their time boundaries because the pioneers in the field began their writing in the early 1940's. The authors were researching and annotating during the year 1991. The literature published during that year was difficult to acquire due to delays in publishing, library acquisition and indexing. Therefore, the authors chose 1990 as the final year for inclusion in this bibliography.

The bibliography is divided into two sections, each containing a subdivision of chapters. The first section includes works focused on theoretical literature in dance/movement therapy. The second section contains chapters focusing specifically on clinical populations. The operational definition of "theoretical" as used for this project is the philosophies and doctrines developed in association with research and practice which shape dance/movement therapy as a psychotherapeutic discipline.

Materials that digress from this definition are not included in this project. Materials selected for inclusion in the clinical practice section are specifically focused on dance/movement therapy with clients. The division of populations reflects the nature of the clinical work of dance/movement therapists and literature. Some of the chapter headings reflect diagnostic categories as dictated by the American Psychiatric Association (1987) standards in the DSM-III-R diagnostic system.

Non-evaluative annotations follow each citation, which relate an encapsulated version of the authors' intent and thesis. For cross-referencing purposes, at the left margin of each citation a number appears chronologically ordering each entry. The literature that is related to more than one population, or provides information on both theoretical and clinical issues, is annotated where the citation appears first alphabetically. A non-annotated second citation appears in relevant population chapters with a cross-referencing number referring the reader back to where the original citation and annotation appear. The symbol (+) appears with the relevant number on the line following the citation. This enables the reader to be referred directly to the citation where the full annotation appears.

In instances when an article or book was published more than once, both citations appear before the annotation. There may be qualitative or quantitative differences in the writings in either source, however, presenting both citations offers the reader research options in securing the material.

Appendix A includes material unavailable to the authors for annotation within the necessary time boundaries of the project. Although the authors' intent for the project was to create a comprehensive annotated theoretical and clinical bibliography of published works in the field, some materials could not be located for annotation. Therefore, Appendix A includes the remainder of citations accumulated in the gathering process.

The following subject areas were accessed by manual and computer searches: arts and humanities, education, medicine, psychology, and social science. Within the category of arts and humanities, manual searches included the Arts and Humanities Index, and the American Humanities Index. Computer searches included the Humanities Citation Index. In education, a manual search was conducted using the Education Index, as well as a computer search using the ERIC system. Within the category of medicine, manual searches included Index Medicus, Quarterly Cumulative Index Medicus, and the Current List of Medical Literature. Computer searches included Medline, EMBASE, and Grateful Med systems. In psychology, the manual search included Psychological Abstracts, and the computer search covered information in the Psych Info system. Within the category of social sciences, two manual searches were completed, covering the Social Science Index and the Social Science Citation Index.

Libraries at the following institutions were utilized to procure material for annotation: Case Western Reserve University, Commission on Mental Health Services at St. Elizabeths Campus, Goucher College, The Library of Congress, The National Library of Medicine at the National Institute of Health, Springfield State Mental Hospital, the University of Maryland, and The Washington Research Library Consortium, which includes: American University, Catholic University of America, Gallaudet University, George Mason University, The George Washington University, Georgetown University, Marymount University, and The University of the District of Columbia. Computer searches by author or title that provided the location of sources were conducted on the Aladin, MCAT and the Grateful Med systems.

After exhausting the resources of Library of Congress, in terms of citation gathering and annotating, the research process expanded to other libraries. To remain organized, the citations were ordered according to the libraries in which they were housed. The researchers spent the necessary time at each library to exhaust the resources housed in that collection before moving on to the next library. Materials unavailable within the necessary boundaries of the project are provided in Appendix A.

The authors became aware of trends in the literature during the research process. Trends included theoretical differences that have emerged in distinct geographical areas, and the growth of the field as it moves from an adjunct therapy to a primary therapy. Another apparent trend was the fluctuating name of the profession and terms used by dance/movement therapists to describe and define their work (e.g., dance/movement therapy, dance therapy, movement therapy, movement psychotherapy, and psychodance). Also discovered was an inconsistency in follow-up of research papers. It appeared that researchers were isolated in their work; if and when a follow-up study was conducted, it was typically written by the original researcher. The growth of psychiatric and psychological theory and vocabulary from 1940 to 1990 produced a pattern of changing and molding to these models in the field of dance/movement therapy.

Finally, several components of the project were restructured to better represent the literature. In order to establish integrity and consistency, the authors made several crucial decisions. The clinical populations section was restructured according to interplay between the DSM-III-R diagnostic system and the multi-faceted work of the dance/movement therapist. To create a consistent and easily readable bibliography, the term dance/movement therapy was chosen for use throughout the project to represent the various labels that currently define the work. It was not the intent of the authors to compromise the integrity and individuality of therapists who choose not to use this term.

As a result of the authors' attempt to organize a large mass of literature while trying to maintain a level of integrity and consistency in the project, much important literature used in the training and practice of dance/movement therapists could not be included within the boundaries of this project. Therefore, the authors foresee that this project could be expanded in several ways. One option would be to create a supplement that would include the clinical and theoretical literature written after 1990. Another option would be to organize dance/movement therapy literature included in Appendix A that fall outside of the boundaries of this project. Other formats could provide supportive dance/movement therapy literature covering non-verbal behavior and communication, movement analysis, literature covering psychological and psychiatric paradigms used in the training and practice of dance/movement therapists, or the history of dance and its anthropological and sociological implications. Any of these formats would be enhanced by a subject or author index. The authors are aware that these constructs are not the only ways in which to organize all of the areas that dance/movement therapy draws upon to create, communicate and document the profession. It is the authors' hope that future researchers will add to this list from their own experience, incorporating new trends and future growth in the field of dance/movement therapy.

SECTION I
THEORETICAL AND RESEARCH MATERIAL

1. Anderson, W. (1977). Dance therapy. In W. Anderson (Ed.), <u>Therapy and the arts: Tools of consciousness</u> (pp. 51-58). New York: Harper & Row.

   The author describes his experience participating in group sessions. The discussion suggests dance/movement therapy as a tool for producing communication, expanding socialization, creating joy and exploring different ways of being.

2. Avstreich, A. K. (1981). The emerging self: Psychoanalytic concepts of self development and their implications for dance therapy. <u>American Journal of Dance Therapy</u>, <u>4</u>(2), 21-32.

   A psychoanalytic view of the psychological birth is presented. The author discusses the implications of the development of the self for theory and practice of dance/movement therapy. Using the developmental model, the author highlights a child's needs and interactions from symbiosis through the separation-individuation process. These include dependency, development of self, togetherness and aloneness, integration of self, spatial needs, the need for mastery and differentiation. The author presents these as the issues of therapy, and gives case examples of work with clients to support these ideas.

3. Baillio, E. (1972). Shall we dance? <u>Journal of Music Therapy</u>, <u>9</u>(1), 37-39.

   The author describes a dance/movement therapy program in a state hospital. The program has three components; the social group structure component for the most profoundly regressed patients focuses on dance as nonverbal communication. The dance as a performance art component is formatted for individual patients who can verbalize but need an outlet for emotions. The dance as physical exercise component uses either a group or individual framework to increase relaxation and coordination, reduce inhibitions and decrease weight.

4 Bainbridge, G., Duddington, A. E., Collingdon, M. & Gardner, C. E. (1953). Dance-mime: A contribution to treatment in psychiatry. <u>Journal of Mental Science</u>, <u>99</u>, 308-314.

An early article suggesting a place for dance and mime in the treatment of psychiatric illness. The authors review ritual in cultural dance from a psychoanalytic paradigm and discuss the use of rhythm with the patient diagnosed with schizophrenia.

5 Bartenieff, I. (1972-73). Dance therapy: A new profession or a rediscovery of an ancient role of the dance. <u>Dance Scope</u>, <u>7</u>(1), 6-18.

The author traces the history of dance/movement therapy through the development of modern dance, to the first pioneers of dance/movement therapy and their philosophies, concluding with the founding and expanding of the American Dance Therapy Association. The author discusses the areas in which practitioners agree and disagree, looking forward to what the field will become.

6 Bartenieff, I. with Lewis, D. (1980). <u>Body movement: Coping with the environment</u>. New York: Gorden and Breach Science Publishers.

One chapter of this book focuses on dance/movement therapy. The author explores this topic by examining the balance between polarities in the work, structure and permissiveness, internal and external experience, subjectivity and objectivity and the self as individual and community member. Bartenieff Fundamentals and Labananalysis are suggested as movement resources.

7 Bennett, R. K. (1982). Sexuality: The foundation of the dance therapy process. In S. Kleinman (Ed.), <u>Sexuality and the Dance</u>, (pp. 1-3). Reston, VA: American Alliance for Health, Physical Education, Recreation, and Dance.

The author suggests that sexuality is the origin of creativity, energy, psychological and physical growth. The article provides a brief examination of sexuality in dance/movement therapy, focusing on therapist sensitivity to their own and others sexuality and a case example of the author's work. The conclusion presents dance/movement therapy as means to express, explore and transform sexual energy from dysfunctional to healthier patterns.

8   Bernstein, P. L. (Ed.). (1979). <u>Eight theoretical approaches in dance/movement therapy</u>. Dubuque, IA: Kendall/Hunt.

Bernstein, P. L. (Ed.). (1986). <u>Theoretical approaches in dance/movement therapy</u> (Vol I). Dubuque, IA: Kendall/Hunt.

The editor provides information on the fundamental theoretical frameworks used in the field. These include: Alderian, Chacian, Gestalt, Jungian, Psychoanalytic, Psychodynamic, Transpersonal-Transformational and Schoop's approach. Chapters are written by pioneers within the field and their students. Clinical examples are given for each framework. The editor concludes the book with a holistic framework that distills and integrates the key material from the major approaches previously discussed, attempting to provide a common conceptual framework for the field.

9   Bernstein, P. L. (Ed.). (1984). <u>Theoretical approaches in dance/movement therapy</u> (Vol II). Dubuque, IA: Kendall/Hunt.

Lewis, P. (Ed.). (1984). <u>Theoretical approaches in dance/movement therapy</u> (Vol. II). Dubuque, IA: Kendall/Hunt.

Section one of this book offers four more theoretical frames of reference in dance/movement therapy to expand Volume One published by the editor (see previous citation). Included are: the methods of Blanche Evan, object relations and self psychology within psychoanalytic and Jungian dance/movement therapy, family therapy in motion; observing, assessing and changing the family dance and experiential movement psychotherapy. In section two, the dance/movement therapy therapeutic process utilizing the phenomenological method is discussed. Explored in this section are: the somatic unconscious and it's relation to the embodied feminine in dance/movement therapy process and the somatic countertransference; the inner pas de deux.

10   Bernstein, P. L. (1985). Embodied transformational images in dance/movement therapy. *Journal of Mental Imagery*, 9(4), 1-8.

The author suggests the principle that change and transformation can only occur as a result of embodied experience. A discussion focuses on dance/movement therapy techniques that facilitate the process of experience and image embodiment. The psychotherapeutic methods explored are guided improvisation, authentic movement from the client, somatic countertransference within the therapist and the client's embodiment of their own archetypal and unconscious images.

11   Bernstein, P. L. (1981). *Theory and methods in dance/movement therapy*. Dubuque, IA: Kendall/Hunt.

The author explores the relationship of developmental theories with the theory of recapitulation of ontogeny to facilitate the creation of adaptive movement patterns in dance/movement therapy. Effects of culture and symbols on movement behavior are also discussed. The appendix includes: a developmental chart that covers Kestenberg's effort-shape components, ego psychology, Jungian analytic psychology and related developmental constellations. A correlational chart compares Gesell, Piaget, effort/shape and developmental theory. Also included is a chart showing the levels of organization for dance/movement therapy, a maladaptive behavior evaluation form and an outline for movement profile.

12   Bernstein, P. L. & Singer, D. L. (Eds.). (1982). *The choreography of object relations*. Keene, NH: Antioch/New England Graduate School.

The work of dance/movement therapists who use object relations theory and self psychology as the foundations in their diagnostic and therapeutic work is presented in this volume. The book is divided into three sections: a theoretical overview, clinical applications and professional applications. In the first section, theoretical overview, the following topics are explored: object relations, self psychology and dance/movement therapy, and the phenomenology of object relations in dance/movement therapy. In the clinical applications section, the topics include: the choreography of facilitating a therapeutic environment, dance/movement therapy with an autistic child, object relations and movement therapy with a developmentally disabled child, the choreography of separation-individuation and movement therapy with narcissistically wounded women. In the concluding section, professional applications, the topic of object relations and the psychoanalytic supervision of dance/movement therapists is explored.

13   Blumberg, S. & Coche, E. (1980). The use of movement in a psychotherapy group. American Journal of Dance Therapy, 3(2), 56-64.

The authors create an exploratory study to test their broad hypothesis that group dance/movement therapy is an effective treatment for psychiatric patients. Subjects are eight patients with psychotic features in a short term hospital. The results show increase in trust, self-disclosure, self-esteem and assertiveness.

14   Bovard-Taylor, A. & Dragonosky, J.E. (1979). Using personal space to develop a working alliance in dance therapy. American Journal of Dance Therapy, 3(1), 51-61.

The authors review literature on personal space, provide clinical application of the concept to creating rapport in dance/movement therapy, and illustrate their application with a case vignette. The authors recommend the following suggestions on the use of space to create a working therapeutic relationship: allow the patient to control and determine proximity to the therapist, allow changes in spacing to occur, respond to patient's comfort level, be aware of cultural, age, sex and developmental issues of space, and be aware of patient's and therapist's spatial needs.

15   Britton, M. (1984). Dance therapist or therapeutic dancer? *Design for Arts in Education*, *86*(4), 4-8.

In this article the author examines the controversy and conflict surrounding the duality of the dance/movement therapist as both artist and therapist. The author describes the ways in which he uses both types of knowledge and experience while working with clients, focusing on choreography within a developmental framework. The author discusses the way in which graduate programs address both movement and psychology within the curriculum to create graduates who are therapists using dance and movement as a healing modality. The article concludes with a discussion of creative art therapists and of how and why they are devalued by the mental health community.

16   Brooks, D., & Stark, A. (1989). The effect of dance/movement therapy on affect - A pilot study. *American Journal of Dance Therapy*, *11*(2), 101-112.

Utilizing hospitalized and non-hospitalized populations, Zuckerman and Lubin's Multiple Affect Adjective Check List (MAACL) was administered to measure hostility, depression and anxiety. The results indicate that dance/movement therapy significantly affected the affect of the participants.

17   Bruno, C. (1981). Applications and implications of "structured analysis of movement sessions" for dance therapy. *The Arts in Psychotherapy*, *8*(2), 127-133.

The author discusses a system called "Structural Analysis of Movement Sessions" as a method of defining, analyzing and describing a group's functioning. This system is then applied to dance/movement therapy as a framework for choosing various techniques, therapist role and props with different diagnostic groups. The populations include adolescents and clients diagnosed with personality disorders and schizophrenia.

18　　　　Bruno, C. (1990). Maintaining a concept of the dance in dance/movement therapy. <u>American Journal of Dance Therapy</u>, <u>12</u>(2), 101-113.

The author follows dance/movement therapy as used within the medical model from the post WWII era to the end of the 1980s'. The author reviews various dance/movement therapeutic approaches and discusses the trend away from the dance in dance/movement therapy.

19　　　　Bunney, J. (1977). Dance therapy. In P. Valletutti and F. Christophs (Eds.), <u>Interdisciplinary approaches to human services</u> (pp. 49-59). Baltimore, MD: University Park Press.

This article proposes to vanquish misunderstandings about the nature of dance/movement therapy as a profession and the training involved in becoming a therapist. The author illuminates the then current state of the following subjects: the goals of dance/movement therapy, clients and settings, equipment, professional training, accreditation of training institutions, registry, research, dance/movement therapy vs. education, interdisciplinary aspects and the time and cost of services.

20　　　　Chace, M. (1960). A note on dance therapy. <u>Group Psychotherapy and Psychodrama</u>, <u>13</u>(3-4), 205.

The author discusses dance/movement therapy as transcending communication barriers and creating community. The author focuses on use of rhythms, simple body dance movement and the circle formation.

21　　　　Chace, M. (1964, July). Dance alone is not enough. <u>Dance Magazine</u>, pp. 46-47, 58.

The author defines dance/movement therapy and offers a framework for the clinical and academic training of the dance/movement therapist, pondering whether dance/movement therapy training should be at the post-graduate level and offering insights into initial clinical training. The author emphasizes the need for clinical and academic training to augment dance training for the well-rounded dance/movement therapist.

22   Chace, M. (1953). Dance as an adjunctive therapy with hospitalized mental patients. <u>Bulletin of the Menninger Clinic</u>, <u>17</u>, 219-225.

The author lays a foundation for dance/movement therapy through a discussion of nonverbal behavior as communication. Examples are provided of author's work as a therapist in terms of setting, the structure of sessions and dance/movement therapy techniques.

23   Chace, M. (1956, June). Dance therapy for the mentally ill. <u>Dance Magazine</u>, pp. 37-39, 58.

The author describes her philosophy of dance/movement therapy. The article begins with observations of dance as innate in human beings, and recommends dance as a means of nonverbal communication and adjunct therapy. The power and use of rhythm is stressed. The therapist's goals presented are to break through patients' isolation and to awaken awareness of the whole self. Important to the session is matching patients' movement style, fluidity of structure and non-dominating leadership. The article closes with a discussion of training for the dance/movement therapist.

24   Chace, M. (1954). Dancing helps patients make initial contacts. <u>Mental Hospitals</u>, <u>5</u>(2), 4-6.

Bringing dance to hospital wards to enrich the daily routine of acutely ill or chronic, regressed patients is the focus of this article. The author hypothesizes that the role of dance may change for patients throughout the course of their hospitalization; that initially, dance can be used for better body control, and as they prepare to leave the hospital, dance can be used as a creative outlet for social contacts. Other issues addressed are the therapist's ability to lay authority aside and allow the emergence of group themes, acceptance of patient interpretations of music and movement, and group development.

25   Chace, M. (1952). Opening doors through dance. *Journal of the American Association for Health, Physical Education and Recreation, 23*(2), 10-11, 34, 39.

Dance and its effects on depressed and psychiatric patients is the focus of this article. The author describes a dance/movement therapy session in terms of waltz, circle formation, movement, conversation, and rhythmic action. The author also explores the actions of the "watchers" on the periphery of the circle formation and considers how they are connected to the action of the group, and when and how to engage them therapeutically. The author concludes by discussing the advantages of the circle formation, as well as how restlessness is expressed in dance.

26   Chaiklin, H. (Ed). (1975). *Marian Chace: Her papers*. Columbia, MD: American Dance Therapy Association.

The editor provides a compilation of documents that reflect the life and work of pioneer Marian Chace. The book is divided into five sections: biographical, published, panel discussions, unpublished and about. It is the intent of the editor to allow the papers to "speak for themselves," and to keep comment and explanation to a minimum. On Ms. Chace's life and creative work, the editor includes a biography, a brief autobiographical statement, some of Ms. Chace's professional notes, notes on her trip to introduce dance/movement therapy in Israel and an outline of a book on dance/movement therapy that Ms. Chace had begun. Topics of Ms. Chace's work include published writings on: her work at St. Elizabeths and Chestnut Lodge Hospitals, rhythm, the use of dance in therapy for the mentally ill, techniques for the use of dance as a group therapy, measurable and intangible aspects of dance sessions, the power of movement with others, movement and personality, and movement communication with children. Previously unpublished materials include: the arts and mental illness, leadership in dance sessions, rhythmic action and body image. The last section, "about," offers two selections about Ms. Chace's personal and professional stature, written by Edith M. Stern and Irmgard Bartenieff, and a poem, "In Memorium - Marian Chace," by Eithne Tabor.

27   Chaiklin, S. (1974). Concepts of dance therapy. *Group Psychotherapy*, 20, 3-4.

The author discusses the basic therapeutic aspects of dance/movement therapy. These include: movement as a tool to communicate and explore emotions, to build and understand relationships with the self and others, to facilitate the body/mind connection and to re-establish the ability to achieve.

28   Chaiklin, S. (1975). Dance therapy. In S. Arieti (Ed.), *American Handbook of Psychiatry* (pp. 701-720). New York: Basic Books.

In this article, the author explores the historical development of dance/movement therapy. Also discussed are psychological and physiological concepts as related to dance/movement therapy, research and movement observation, goals and structure of dance/movement therapy and description of a group session. Theoretical frameworks for the following populations are offered: autism, neuroses and schizophrenia.

29   Chaiklin, S. (1977). Defining therapeutic goals. *American Journal of Dance Therapy*, 1(1), 25-29.

The author presents the need for a clear conceptual framework and a systematized base of knowledge from which client referral, treatment approaches and goals can be defined and executed in dance/movement therapy. The author explores basic therapeutic assumptions, such as the gathering of useful information for treatment, structure of the treatment session, treatment goals and promoting behavioral change as they pertain to dance/movement therapy as a psychotherapeutic discipline. A brief case example outlines the author's experience in gathering diagnostic material, movement observations, treatment goals and the initial therapeutic process.

30   Costonis, M. N. (Ed.). (1978). *Therapy in Motion*. Urbana-Champaign, IL: University of Illinois Press.

This book consists of a collection of writings that focus on four areas of study: communicating through expressive movement, expanding the movement repertoire, enhancing body awareness and the creative "interface" which presents samples of therapists' interaction styles. Clinical populations include autism and schizophrenia. The text includes an extensive bibliography.

31   Creamer, N. (1983). The silent language: Basic principles of movement/dance therapy for the non-movement therapist. *Journal of Group Psychotherapy, Psychodrama and Sociometry*, *36*(2), 55-60.

The author reviews a didactic and experiential workshop created for the non-dance/movement therapist. Workshop participants took part in a dance/movement therapy session and explored the role of mixed messages (e.g. verbal and non-verbal) in client/therapist interactions. A psychodrama/dance/movement therapy session in which participants explored ways of integrating verbal and non-verbal messages is discussed.

32   Dosamantes, E. (1990). Movement and psychodynamic pattern changes in long term dance/movement therapy groups. *American Journal of Dance Therapy*, *12*(1), 27-44.

An experiment in which the author examines expected changes of four pre-selected movement and psychodynamic variables: individual movement style, interpersonal movement style, individual psychodynamics and object relations, and functions served by the therapist. The study was conducted over the course of two years. Subjects include 22 graduate students in dance/movement therapy. The results indicate movement and psychodynamic changes in both individual and interactional movement styles.

33 Dosamantes-Alperson, E. (1974). Carrying experiencing forward through authentic body movement. *Psychotherapy: Theory, Research and Practice*, *11*(3), 211-215.

Dosamantes-Alperson, E. (1976). Carrying experiencing forward through authentic body movement. In Banet, A.G. (Ed.). *Creative psychotherapy: A sourcebook*. LaJolla, CA: University Press Association.

Dance/movement therapy is discussed as a transformational process in which clients make contact with their own experiencing, and change energy and body movement into imagery and verbal symbols. The author suggests that this process of experiencing organic movement creates change by unblocking old patterns, exploring new ones and allowing insight into previously unresolved issues.

34 Dosamantes-Alperson, E. (1980). Dance/movement therapy: An Emerging profession. *Journal of Energy Medicine*, *1*(1), 114-119.

The author introduces dance/movement therapy in terms of the historical value of dance, the American Dance Therapy Association, therapist training and the variety of potential populations. Goals shared with verbal therapies are mentioned (e.g., increased kinesthetic awareness and spontaneity). The author defines her approach as experiential, following Gendlin's experiential philosophy and theory. Using examples from the authors work with clients, she describes her own style of dance/movement therapy. Research and evaluation are suggested as means to promote and strengthen the field.

35 Dosamantes-Alperson, E. (1981). Experiencing in movement psychotherapy. *American Journal of Dance Therapy*, *4*(2), 33-45.

The author discusses the act of experiencing in relation to successful psychotherapy. The methods suggested for facilitating experiencing in dance/movement therapy sessions include focusing on bodily-felt experiences, embodying conflict and exploring personal and interactional space.

36   Dosamantes-Alperson, E. (1977). Experiential movement psychotherapy. <u>American Journal of Dance Therapy</u>, <u>1</u>(1), 8-12.

The author describes the theories and methods of experiential movement psychotherapy and discusses three therapist blocks that inhibit therapeutic process: fear of differences, fear of being perceived as fallible and fear of client fragility.

37   Dosamantes-Alperson, E. (1977). Nonverbal and verbal integration. In W. Anderson (Ed.), <u>Therapy and the arts: Tools of consciousness</u> (pp. 59-66). New York: Harper & Row.

An investigation is presented of the strengths and weaknesses of both verbal therapy and dance/movement therapy. Strengths of verbalization include feeling validation by another, verbal sharing, clarification of feelings and perceptions, and externalizing and owning personal reactions. The author suggests knowing the self as the source of experience, awareness of felt-experience, outward expression of inner attitude as the strengths of movement. The article concludes with the author's recommendation of coupling authentic verbalization in dance/movement therapy sessions to create integrated change.

38   Dosamantes-Alperson, E. (1974). The creation of meaning through body movement. In A. I. Rabin (Ed.), <u>Clinical psychology: Issues of the seventies</u>. (pp. 156-165). E. Lansing, MI: Michigan State University Press.

The author surveys pragmatic and humanistic approaches in psychotherapy, and examines trends that have emerged from the humanist ideology. Exploring and applying to dance/movement therapy the work of theorists Gendlin, Ornstein and Laing, the author discusses authentic movement in dance/movement therapy as a felt level of experiencing that precedes the conceptual-verbal level of experiencing.

39   Dosamantes-Alperson, E. (1981). The interaction between movement and imagery in experiential movement psychotherapy. *Psychotherapy: Theory, Research and Practice*, *18*(2), 266-271.

The author describes the process of combining imagery and movement during dance/movement therapy sessions to increase self knowledge and produce conflict resolution. The process promotes contacting bodily felt experiences, transforming these experiences into visual symbols, addressing conflicts in the movement-image interaction. General principles for enhancing the experience are suggested including releasing tensions, focusing on the body, creating a movement symbol interaction, following the interaction and verbalizing the experience.

40   Dosamantes-Alperson, E. (1979). The intrapsychic and interpersonal in movement psychotherapy. *American Journal of Dance Therapy*, *3*(1), 20-31.

The author explores the dance/movement therapist's responsibilities to offer an opportunity for clients to integrate internal and external experience in relation to intrapsychic and interpersonal events. The author suggests frameworks for facilitating the receptive mode (e.g., contacting bodily-felt experiencing, creating a movement-imagery intervention) and the action mode (e.g., creating a safe environment, and encouraging the expansion of the client's movement vocabulary). Clinical examples are cited to demonstrate these techniques.

41   Dosamantes-Alperson, E. (1987). Transference and countertransference issues in movement psychotherapy. *The Arts in Psychotherapy*, *14*(3), 209-214.

The author discusses transference and countertransference as potential therapeutic instruments for the psychoanalytically-trained movement therapist. The author includes a section that discusses defensive strategies used by therapists to avoid unpleasant countertransference reactions.

42   Dosamantes-Alperson, E. (1982-83). Working with internalized relationships through a kinesthetic and kinetic imagery process. *Imagination, Cognition and Personality*, *2*(4), 333-343.

The author distinguishes traditional verbal psychotherapy from experiential movement psychotherapy and offers movement action and imagery as a rationale in processing unconscious material for the derivation of personal meaning from experiencing. A case illustration exploring the use of a kinetic imagery process in which the client retrieves unconscious aspects of internalized relationships is included.

43   Dosamantes-Alperson, E. & Merrill, N. (1980). Growth effects of experiential movement psychotherapy. *Psychotherapy: Theory, Research and Practice*, *17*(1), 63-38.

The authors examine claims of change from the clinical setting, in this controlled experiment. The effects of experiential movement psychotherapy are measured in terms of physical self-acceptance and self-actualization. The tools used to measure change are Shostrom's Personal Orientation Inventory, Secord-Jourards Body-Cathexis Scale, and Dosamantes-Alperson's Expressive Movement Scale. The experimental procedure consisted of twice-weekly dance/movement therapy sessions one and one half hours long each, for a total of 16 sessions. Results show a significant increase in both physical body acceptance and self-actualization.

44   Duggan, D. (1981). Dance therapy. In R. Corsini (Ed.), *Innovative Psychotherapies*, (pp. 229-240). New York: Wiley & Sons.

This article is an introduction to dance/movement therapy emphasizing the history of the profession, the then current status of the field, the author's theoretical framework, methodologies used by therapists, application in terms of client populations and a case study of her work with a neurotic woman in group dance/movement therapy. In the theoretical section, the author describes a developmental framework. She suggests dance/movement therapy as an integrative form of communication that affects many parts of self through the process of experiencing, as well as expands the repertoire of adaptive responses. The methodology section includes a discussion of the role of effort/shape, mirroring, directive and non-directive approaches, structure, props and verbalization.

45 Ellis, R. W. & Wersen, K. (1958, August). Motion & emotion: Questions and answers about dance therapy for the mentally ill. <u>Dance Magazine</u>, pp. 48-51, 73.

The authors discuss the differences between dance/movement therapy, other therapies and modern dance, offering their definition of dance/movement therapy. The authors further explore the goals of a dance/movement therapy session, qualification and training for the dance/movement therapist and speculations about the future of dance/movement therapy. The authors state that it is "the far-sighted dancer interested in his fellow men that will investigate this new and exciting area."

46 Espenak, L. (1981). <u>Dance therapy: Theory and application</u>. Springfield, IL: Thomas.

The author presents an explanatory and instructive description of dance/movement therapy. The author incorporates psychomotor theory into dance/movement therapy in terms of theory, diagnosis and evaluation, treatment and expressive group interaction. Populations discussed include autism, mental retardation, neuroses and schizophrenia. Appendices provide lists of suggested films, music and readings.

47 Espenak, L. (1970). Movement diagnostic tests and the inherent laws governing their use in treatment: An aid in detecting the lifestyle. <u>Individual Psychologist</u>, <u>7</u>(1), 8-13.

Working within an Adlerian framework, the author relates a "working-method" for assessing the dynamic possibilities inherent in individual patients. Six Movement Diagnostic Tests that measure positive and negative aspects of personality are included. They are: Body Image, Emotional State (Spatial Relationships), Degree of

Dynamic Drive (Force Adjustment), Control of Dynamic Drive (Rhythm, Time Concepts), Coordination (Body Awareness and Locomotion), Endurance (Constancy) and Physical Courage (Anxiety States).

48 Feder, E. & Feder, B. (1977). Dance Therapy. <u>Psychology Today</u>, <u>10</u>(9), 76-80.

Dance/movement therapy is discussed in terms of it's ability to relieve muscular tension, interpret nonverbal communication and discover muscle memory. The author gives examples of group sessions from an outpatient clinic and examples of individual therapy at a day care center for children diagnosed with autism.

49 Feder, E. & Feder, B. (1981). <u>The expressive arts therapies</u>. Englewood Cliffs, NJ: Prentice-Hall.

One chapter of this book focuses on dance/movement therapy. Areas discussed by the authors include research, diagnosis, effort/shape, the therapeutic use of movement and current issues within the field. Case examples supporting the use of dance/movement therapy examine the following populations: autism, neuroses and schizophrenia.

50 Froehlich, M. A. (1985). An annotated bibliography for the creative arts therapies. <u>Journal of Music Therapy</u>, <u>2</u>(4), 218-226.

The bibliography covers books written in the fields of art, dance/movement, drama and puppet therapy. Eleven dance/movement therapy books are included, spanning 1968-1978. The annotations are evaluative and provide description of topics covered within each book.

51 Goodill, S. & Leatherbee, T. (Eds.). (1984). <u>A primer for assessment and evaluation in dance/movement therapy</u>. Philadelphia, PA: Hahnemann University.

A collection of writings that provide methods and frameworks that integrate biological, cognitive, emotional and creative phenomena in movement assessment and evaluation. Case examples include childhood disorders, geriatrics, neuroses and schizophrenia.

52 Hanna, J. L. (1978). African dance: Some implications for dance therapy. <u>American Journal of Dance Therapy</u>, <u>2</u>(1), 3-15.

This article draws upon the author's study of Nigeria's Ukabala dance-plays. The author explores three main areas: the relationship of dance to the individual and society, psychobiological bases of dance and forms expressing meaning in movement. The author developed a "semantic grid" from study that can be transferrable to dance/movement therapy for diagnosing problems and measuring change.

53 Hanna, J. L. (1988). <u>Dance and Stress</u>. New York: AMS Press.

In a chapter describing dance/movement therapy, the author describes dance/movement therapy as means to induce and dissipate stress. The author presents several theoretical approaches including Freudian, Jungian, Reichian, Gestalt-phenomenological, Sullivan's interpersonal theory of personality, learning theory, psychomotor developmental theory and group therapy theory. The author places emphasis on the theory of group psychotherapy. Clinical examples from the populations of geriatrics and childhood disorders are given to support the author's ideas that dance/movement therapy can produce as well as reduce stress.

54 Harris, J. & Beers, J. (1974). <u>Bibliography on dance therapy</u>. Columbia, MD: American Dance Therapy Association.

The authors arrange this bibliography by topic. Those presented are: the theory, practice and research of dance/movement therapy, movement fundamentals, non-verbal communication, body image, other psychotherapeutic approaches to treatment, the child, creativity, art, education and the psychic experience, group and group dynamics, selected readings in psychology, psychiatry, and supportive literary and cultural material. The entries span the time period of early 1940's to early 1970's. No unpublished materials are included. A film list is presented. Evaluative annotations are provided for some entries.

55 Hood, C. C. (1959). Challenge of dance therapy. *Journal of Health, Physical Education and Recreation*, 30, 17-18.

The author presents the results of the American Association of Health, Physical Education and Recreation (AAHPER) Dance/Movement Therapy Study Committee investigation into the current activities in the field. The discussion is drawn from information gathered from questionnaires answered by dance/movement therapists, and psychiatrists or administrators. Information covered includes a definition of dance/movement therapy, training of therapists and opportunities in the field.

56 Johnson, D. R., Sandel, S. L. & Eicher, V. (1983). Structural aspects of group leadership styles. *American Journal of Dance Therapy*, 6, 17-31.

The authors discuss the therapist as a leader in group dance/movement therapy sessions in terms of management functions. These functions include maintaining the external group boundary, controlling the level of complexity in group tasks, overseeing and containing the group interaction, and tolerating ambiguity and uncertainty. Three dance/movement therapists are analyzed in terms of management functions and suggestions are given for increasing the therapist's effectiveness.

57 Kaveler, S. & Riess, B. F. (1977). Dance therapy. *Transnational Mental Health Research Newsletter*, 19(1), 2-5.

The authors provide a general definition of dance/movement therapy. An introduction is given about work with various populations including patients with schizophrenia, clients with neuroses and children with either emotional disturbances and/or learning disabilities. Dance/movement therapy is suggested as an ancillary tool to verbal psychotherapies.

58   Keleher, C. G. (1956). Modern dance as mental therapy. *Dance Observer, 23*(3), 37.

This article contains a description of dance/movement therapy as effective in stimulating change in behavior with psychiatric populations. It is suggested that there is a need for a greater number of staff in the mental health field.

59   Koch, N. S. (1984). Content analysis of leadership variables in dance therapy. *American Journal of Dance Therapy, 7*, 58-75.

Dance/movement therapy leadership variables are defined and analyzed in this content analysis study. The author defines leadership content with the following selected categories: terminology describing the dance/movement therapist, personality variables, roles, goals and approaches to treatment. The following books were selected by the author for their historical perspective, spanning 34 years of development in the field: *Marian Chace: Her papers* (1975), *Dance therapy: Focus on dance VII* (1974) and *Eight theoretical approaches to dance/movement therapy* (1979).

60   Kuettel, T. J. (1982). Affective change in dance therapy. *American Journal of Dance Therapy, 5*, 56-64.

The author conducts two pilot studies in which the effect of dance/movement therapy on affect is measured. The hypotheses are that subjects in one hour of dance/movement therapy would express more affect than subjects in a control group, and that subjects receiving 45 minutes of dance/movement therapy would report more affect than subjects receiving a 45 minute T-group. The subjects include female nursing and occupational therapy students who completed pretest and posttest Feelings Questionnaire for each dance/movement therapy session. On scores for erotized affection, anxious, and somatic distress, as well as confident, inhibited and depressed affect, the results supported the hypotheses.

61   Kuettel, T. J. (1983). Professional productivity among registered dance therapists. <u>American Journal of Dance Therapy</u>, <u>6</u>, 74-90.

The author provides an examination into the overall productivity of dance/movement therapists. The research yields productivity information in reference to educational differences, professional activities, published materials and presentations. The author assesses differences between therapists who hold Ph.D.'s and two types of master's degrees. The results provide information on the interaction between the above listed variables in terms of therapist productivity.

62   Leatherbee, T. (1979). Interfaces of creativity: A mini-symposium. <u>Art Psychotherapy</u>, <u>6</u>(3), 147.

The author proposes both art and dance as therapeutic modalities that may strengthen defenses and facilitate insight. Creativity is described as the expression and result of increased internal tension. The author suggests developing a dialogue between art and dance/movement therapists on treatment teams to discuss the effectiveness of these creative arts therapies, and to broaden understanding of patients as they express themselves in different modalities.

63   Leatherbee, T. & Wood, S. (Eds.). (1985). <u>A primer for theoretical models and clinical work in dance/movement therapy</u>. Philadelphia, PA: Hahnemann University Medical College.

A book in which specific topics and models of theoretical and practical thought in the field of dance/movement therapy are introduced. The editors propose that this book be used as textbook for beginning students. Areas covered include: minimalistic approach with a child diagnosed with a severe disturbance, individual sessions with adolescents diagnosed with emotional disturbances and learning disabilities, sessions with children and their families, groups with young adults diagnosed with mental retardation, short-term inpatient treatment, dance/movement therapy with adult inpatients, bio-psycho-social framework, the use of humor a partial hospital setting, work with normal adult population, beginning and executing dance/movement therapy with boarding school population, work with geriatrics and an approach to treatment of children with emotional disturbances.

64 Lefco, H. (1974). <u>Dance therapy: Narrative case histories of therapy sessions with six patients</u>. Chicago, IL: Nelson-Hall.

The author recounts work with six inpatients participating in a long-term dance/movement therapy group. Aspects of the work include: transference and countertransference, therapist boundaries and group dynamics.

65 Levy, F. J. (1988). <u>Dance/movement therapy: A healing art</u>. Reston, VA: American Alliance for Health, Physical Education, Recreation and Dance.

The author outlines the field's growth, focusing on pioneers of dance/movement therapy and their work. Major pioneers covered include Irmgard Bartenieff, Marian Chace, Liljian Espenak, Blanche Evan, Alma Hawkins, Trudi Schoop and Mary Whitehouse. Populations include: autism, childhood disorders, eating disorders, geriatrics, neuroses, special needs, schizophrenia and sexual abuse.

66 Levy, F. J. (1979). Psychodramatic movement therapy: A sorting out process. <u>American Journal of Dance Therapy</u>, <u>3</u>(1), 32-42.

Psychodrama and dance/movement therapy are combined to create fuller therapeutic experience. The author suggests the use of dance/movement therapy techniques to begin sessions and develop material, and psychodramatic structures for expression of affect and working through thematic material.

67   Levy, F. J. (1988). The evolution of modern dance therapy. *Journal of Physical Education, Recreation and Dance*, *59*(5), 34-41.

The author explores dance in culture, the evolution of modern dance and the growth of dance therapy as a psychotherapeutic field. The transition of pioneers in dance/movement therapy from modern dancers to dance/movement therapists is also discussed.

68   Mason, K. C. (Ed.). (1974). Dance therapy. *Focus on Dance VII*, 72. Washington, D.C.: American Alliance for Health, Physical Education and Recreation.

The editor presents dance/movement therapy as an emerging profession through a compilation of material from many authors that support the editor's thesis. The variety of topics covered are organized into these general categories: an introduction to dance/movement therapy, philosophy and methods, techniques for research and observation, client populations, training and professional status.

69   May, R. (1941). Modern dancing as a therapy for the mentally ill. *Occupational Therapy and Rehabilitation*, *20*, 101-106.

Based on psychoanalytic theory, the author promotes the use of modern dance as therapy. The author recommends dance/movement therapy as vehicle for working through disturbances in the aggressive and erotic drives. A discussion of the limits of the therapy is included.

70   McCarthy, H. (1973). The use of the draw-a-person test to evaluate a dance therapy program. *Journal of Music Therapy*, *10*(3), 141-155.

This study examines dance/movement therapy's power to promote integration and internalization of body image and personal identity. Draw-a-person tests were used to evaluate change in adult psychiatric patients involved in dance/movement therapy over a two month period. Results demonstrated positive therapeutic changes in body image and feelings of personal identity.

71   McNiff, S. (1981). The arts and psychotherapy. Springfield, IL: Thomas.

The author offers one chapter examining the use of dance and movement within expressive arts therapies. In the chapter, the author describes dance in relation to the other arts, and the history of the mind/body split. In the article, the author's personal experience as expressive art therapist with clients using dance/movement therapy techniques is presented.

72   Milberg, D. B. (1977). Directions for research in dance/movement therapy. American Journal of Dance Therapy, 1(2), 14-17.

The author presents the position that dance/movement therapy must, through research, broaden it's exposure to the larger professional community. Three types of scientific research, descriptive, dynamic, and therapeutic, are discussed by author as they pertain to testing hypotheses within the field of dance/movement therapy. The author offers a description and critique of a typical research scenario in dance/movement therapy, describing factors of internal and external validity, correlation and causal relationships, and verifying constructs.

73   Mitchell, J. D. (1987). Dance/movement therapy in a changing health care system. American Journal of Dance Therapy, 10, 4-10.

The author provides information on the changing health care system. He predicts potential issues and prescribes strategies for the field of dance/movement therapy in order to deal with the coming changes. Suggestions include: focusing on work with special needs and geriatric populations, increasing diversity of populations that students study in graduate school and joining creative arts associations to face the future health care system together.

74 North, M. (1972). <u>Personality assessment through movement</u>. Boston, MA: Plays, Inc.

In two chapters of this book, the author discusses dance/movement therapy. The first is an individual case study illustrating a client's characteristic movements and how dance/movement therapy coupled with movement assessment can facilitate change in a person's movement style and enhance overall health. In the other, the author discusses group therapy in terms of structured and non-structured movement sessions, group relationships and the value of group movement.

75 Peterson, B. & Cameron, C. (1978). Preparing high anxiety patients for psychotherapy through body therapy. <u>Journal of Contemporary Psychotherapy</u>, <u>9</u>(2), 171-177.

The hypothesis is presented that dance/movement therapy will decrease anxiety experienced by patients before traditional verbal psychotherapy. A population of psychiatric patients described as suffering from high anxiety are divided into an experimental group of 11 subjects and a control group of 10 subjects. The subjects receiving the experimental condition participated in dance/movement therapy for one and one-half hours weekly for sixteen weeks. The control group receives none. The Taylor Manifest Anxiety Scale, the Minnesota Multiphasic Personality Inventory, and the galvanic skin response test are used to measure anxiety. Mixed results show that anxiety is not significantly reduced, but participants ability to control anxiety is enhanced.

76 Pierpont, M. (1979, February). The annual conference of the American Dance Therapy Association: At a crossing point. <u>Dance Magazine</u>, pp. 88-90.

The author offers overall view of the conference and discusses the different influences emerging in dance/movement therapy on the East Coast (e.g., Chace) and the West Coast (e.g., Jung). The author suggests that dance/movement therapy is in the struggle of adolescence and desires validation by other mental health professionals and the psychiatric community. The influences and trends in dance/movement therapy are followed regionally examining: theoretical constructs, the types of establishments and populations with which dance/movement therapists typically work.

77   Puttock, D. (1972). Dance therapy. <u>Nursing Times</u>, <u>68</u>(31), 960-961.

The author begins with a definition of dance/movement therapy and offers insights on dance as a diagnostic, cathartic and therapeutic tool. A history of dance/movement therapy in the United States and the United Kingdom is explored, with a brief discussion of Chace, Laban, Steiner and Dalcroze. The article concludes with a discussion of prospects and limitations for dance/movement therapy in England.

78   Razy, V. (1970). Dance therapy in a community mental health center. <u>Impulse</u>, (Suppl.), 71-75.

Dance/movement therapy is suggested as a treatment approach that will reinforce patient's motivation to change. The author outlines a plan for developing, initiating and maintaining a dance/movement therapy program. The author presents information regarding: the initiating the program, what to look for in a dance/movement therapist, a session's progression, potential problems (e.g., patients from different cultural backgrounds, gender/dance stereotypes and resistance) and the development of an outpatient program. A dance/movement therapy progress report and referral form are included.

79   Riess, B. F. (1969). Developments in dance therapy. <u>Current Psychiatric Therapies</u>, <u>9</u>, 195-201.

An early article in which the author reviews dance and human movement as expression, focusing on the work of Marian Chace and Trudi Schoop. Also mentioned is the use of rhythm in dance/movement therapy, which includes a case example.

80   Robbins, A. (1980). <u>Expressive therapy: A creative arts approach to depth-oriented treatment</u>. New York: Human Sciences Press.

This book includes two chapters that are related to dance/movement therapy. One presents a comparative discussion of art and dance as treatment modalities. The other is a description of the integration of movement and psychoanalytic technique through an examination of dance/movement therapy as a primary intervention and through the presentation of a case study.

81   Rosen, E. (1974). <u>Dance in psychotherapy</u>. New York: Dance Horizons.

The author hypothesizes that dance/movement therapy is rehabilitative in terms of withdrawal from reality, and will enable and enhance the re-socialization process for persons with psychotic illness. A study is presented that explores the value of dance/movement therapy with institutionalized patients with psychotic disturbances. Clinical material from two dance/movement therapy programs is discussed, including information on group process and individual clinical vignettes. Programs were organized as follows: one group of patients from a back ward, meeting weekly for one hour for four months; one group from an open ward meeting weekly for one hour and one-half; and one group of patients diagnosed with schizophrenia meeting twice weekly for one hour. The author's tentative findings, although non-generalizable, suggest techniques that support her hypothesis.

82   Russell, R. W. (1970). The Wisconsin dance idea: Tribute from a movement therapist. <u>Impulse</u>, (Suppl.), 68-70.

The author describes dance/movement therapy. The basic goals discussed in this article include raising body awareness, kinesthetic response, strengthening the ego, enlarging the movement vocabulary and developing identity. Time, space and force are presented as the major therapeutic tools available to the dance/movement therapist.

83   Sandel, S. L. (1975). Integrating dance therapy into treatment. <u>Hospital and Community Psychiatry</u>, <u>26</u>(7), 439-441.

An article in which the author explores the process of defining therapeutic goals of dance/movement therapy with patients and with the treatment team. The process culminates in the clarification of goals and values within the dance/movement therapy groups.

84   Sandel, S. L. & Johnson, D. R. (1977). Structured analysis of group movement sessions: Preliminary research. <u>American Journal of Dance Therapy</u>, <u>1</u>(2), 32-36.

The authors create a system for describing the events of a group therapy session as well as the group's level of functioning. The system has three basic dimensions for defining patterns that groups form. They are task, space, and role. These basic dimensions combine into 46 types of structures. The authors suggest a system to address diagnosis, level of group development, therapist approach, and specific techniques. Examples of system use in analyzing dance/movement therapy sessions are given.

85   Schlichter, J. R. (1970). Sequence: Psychodance 1964. <u>Impulse</u>, (Suppl.), 76-77.

The author promotes dance as a form of psychotherapy. Potential methods are provided including body level warm-up, mirroring, symbolism, fantasy and pantomime. The article concludes with the suggestion that dance/movement therapy works in the present, addressing the complexities of reality and fantasy through body action.

86   Schmais, C. (1977). Dance therapy as a career. <u>Journal of Physical Education and Recreation</u>, <u>48</u>(5), 38.

In describing dance/movement therapy as a career, the author discusses the skills dancers must bring with them to become therapists (e.g., understanding of symbolic movement and body awareness). Education beyond dance classes and internships are highlighted as important for shaping a dancer into a clinician.

87   Schmais, C. (1967). Dance therapy as a profession. <u>Journal of Health, Physical Education and Recreation</u>, <u>38</u>(1), 63-64.

The author discusses the process that led to the first meeting of the American Dance Therapy Association on October 29, 1966. The article continues with the author urging a dialogue between dance/movement therapy and other professions and stating the need for formalized academic training in the field. The author concludes by suggesting that since dance/movement therapy's "birth pangs" are over, it is time to establish newsletters, workshops and seminars in the field.

88   Schmais, C. (1981). Group development and group formation in dance therapy. <u>The Arts in Psychotherapy</u>, <u>8</u>(2), 103-107.

The author describes the developmental stages of a group in terms of themes and task progression including warmup, development and closure. This overview describes the therapist/client interaction at each developmental stage. The group formations discussed include a single line, a parallel line, a clump, a cluster and scattered formations.

89   Schmais, C. (1985). Healing processes in group dance therapy. <u>American Journal of Dance Therapy</u>, <u>8</u>, 17-36.

The focus of this article is on the curative factors in dance/movement therapy. The author reviews theories on the therapeutic factors of verbal psychotherapy and formulates a list of the transformational elements of dance/movement therapy. These are synchrony, expression, rhythm, vitalization, cohesion, education and symbolism. Each element is defined and described in terms of clinical work.

90 Schmais, C. (1976). What is dance therapy? *Journal of Health, Physical Education and Recreation, 47*(1), 39.

The author defines fundamental differences in the roles, methods and techniques of dance/movement therapists and dance teachers. The role of the dance/movement therapist is described as focusing on emotional problems with clients, while the role of the dance teacher is to know and teach a technique (e.g., modern, ballet). Also explored is the intentional therapeutic intervention of the dance/movement therapist based on the therapeutic relationship to facilitate psychic change, which differs from the psychic benefits one may reap in a dance class.

91 Schmais, C. & Felber, D. J. (1977). Dance therapy process analysis: A method for observing and analyzing a dance therapy group. *American Journal of Dance Therapy, 1*(2), 18-25.

The authors suggest combining traditional research strategies with current technologies of film and video to facilitate a greater understanding of the work of dance/movement therapists. A seven member adolescent group from a psychiatric hospital was videotaped and the following parameters were analyzed for the purpose of this study: musical stops and starts, initiations, vocalizations, touch, synchronous movement, rhythmic synchrony, effort synchrony, spatial synchrony, sagittal movement and small group formations. Upon analysis of data, the authors speculate that a large amount of touch can reflect comfort, dependency and trust, and that observing film is an effective method of measuring a group's synchrony or non-synchrony.

92 Schmais, C. & White, E. Q. (1986). Introduction to dance therapy. *American Journal of Dance Therapy, 9*, 23-30.

This article relates introductory information about dance/movement therapy. The authors highlight the origins of the profession, current usage, what dance/movement therapy is and what it does and the necessary attributes and experiences of dance/movement therapists.

93 Schuster, K. (1978). Dance therapy: Moving with a beat - toward health. <u>Physician and Sportsmedicine</u>, <u>6</u>(12), 95-98.

  An overview of the work of Miriam R. Berger at the Bronx Psychiatric Hospital is outlined in this general article. The author provides information about Berger's philosophy of the program; that dance/movement therapy "attempts to expand [the patients'] use of time, weight and space, and in so doing, expand their feelings." The article concludes with a general description of dance/movement therapy sessions for chronic psychiatric and special needs populations.

94 Seigel, M. B. (1969, January). Describing an elephant. <u>Dance Magazine</u>, pp. 92-93.

  This article presents a description of a workshop co-sponsored by the Committee on Research in Dance, the American Dance Therapy Association and the Postgraduate Center for Mental Health. The aim of this one day conference examines research potentials in the field. The author relates the ideas presented by a variety of movement specialists, psychiatrists and psychologists about researching in the field. These ideas are formulated after having viewed video tapes dance/movement therapy sessions. The issues that resulted from those examinations and discussions include defining the work of the dance/movement therapist, exploring research and exploring various approaches within the field.

95 Serlin, L. (1977). Portrait of Karen: A gestalt-phenomenological approach to movement therapy. <u>Journal of Contemporary Psychotherapy</u>, <u>8</u>(2), 145-152.

  The author presents a discussion of her style of working, the gestalt-phenomenological approach to dance/movement therapy. The article focuses on a case study through which the author weaves theoretical material. The underlying concepts in the author's work are emphasizing awareness, excitement, and involvement (especially responsibility and contact) in the moment-to-moment process of living.

96   Shuman, B. (1973). Dance therapy for the emotionally disturbed. <u>Journal of Health, Physical Education and Recreation</u>, <u>44</u>(7), 61-62.

This introductory article defines basic dance/movement therapy objectives and methods. The objectives and goals as stated by the author are behavioral change, catharsis, the release and relaxation of body tension and self awareness. The dance/movement therapy methods are described as empathy, rhythm, props and improvisation to facilitate growth and self awareness.

97   Siegel, E. V. (1972). About Emily: A movement therapist responds. <u>Voices: The Art and Science of Psychotherapy</u>, <u>8</u>(2), 44-46.

The author gives a narrative description of her own thoughts and feelings as a dance/movement therapist while in her first session with this client. The description focuses on transference, countertransference, physical feelings, emotions and thoughts about the client's experience including: relationship, fears and goals.

98   Siegel, E. V. (1984). <u>Dance/movement therapy: Mirror of ourselves: The psychoanalytic approach</u>. New York: Human Sciences Press.

Psychoanalytic and developmental theories are applied to what the author labels the ego-psychoanalytic approach in dance/movement therapy. From this perspective, the author discusses motility and the ego, the unity of body and mind, human development and transference and countertransference. The case examples include author's work with the following populations: autism, borderline personality disorder, elective mutism, obsessive-compulsive disorder and schizophrenia.

99   Siegel, E. V. (1981). In search of pure perception: An attempt to apply Merleau-Ponty's concepts of sense experiences to psychoanalytically oriented movement therapy. The Arts in Psychotherapy, 3(4), 201-205.

The author explores Merleau-Ponty's theories of perception. Through movement and sensation-oriented experientials, including dancing a color or drawing a piece of music, the author examines the interplay between the senses. The author concludes that reaching the level of sensing can play large part in overcoming defenses.

100   Siegel, E. V. (1973). Movement therapy as a psychotherapeutic tool. Journal of the American Psychoanalytic Association, 21(2), 333-343.

The author creates a rationale for dance/movement therapy as a valid form of psychotherapy. Examples are given from a variety of clinical situations and populations.

101   Siegel, E. V. (1970). Psyche and soma: Movement therapy. Voices: The Art and Science of Psychotherapy, 6, 29-32.

The author defines dance/movement therapy in terms of an ego-analytic framework. The author investigates the integration of body and mind, catharsis and insight gained from regression, client's natural, habitual movement patterns and improvisation as integral parts of the dance/movement therapy process. Examples are given of everyday movement (e.g., pitching a baseball, shaking hands) that communicate unconscious material.

102   Silberman, L. (Ed.). (1981). Dance therapy bibliography, 1981. Columbia, MD: American Dance Therapy Association.

The intent of this bibliography is to compile an exclusive, comprehensive listing of dance/movement therapy literature to date. This bibliography is divided into the following sections: clinical and theoretical dance/movement therapy, early writings on the therapeutic value of movement, research studies on dance/movement therapy, unpublished theses and dissertations and films and selected videotapes.

103   Smallwood, J. (1978). Dance therapy and the transcendent function. <u>American Journal of Dance Therapy</u>, 2(1), 16-23.

The author relates the therapeutic aspects of dance/movement therapy to the Jungian concepts of transcendent function and active imagination. Case examples focusing on the emergence of unconscious material through movement are included.

104   Stark, A. (1987, November). American Dance Therapy Association, A kinesthetic approach. <u>Dance Magazine</u>, pp. 56-57.

While recounting the theoretical basis and goals of dance/movement therapy, the author discusses body awareness and kinesthetic sense as a basis for emotional awareness and response. Included is a brief case example that illustrates self awareness through movement interaction. The author also addresses the history of the profession, the therapeutic process and dance/movement therapy training.

105   Stark, A. (1980). The evolution of professional training in the A.D.T.A. <u>American Journal of Dance Therapy</u>, 3(2), 12-19.

The author describes the education and professional training of dance/movement therapists from the pioneers in the field through then current educational guidelines and training requirements of the American Dance Therapy Association. The author divides this history into the following evolutionary stages: early training in dance/movement therapy, the development of a registry, and graduate training.

106   Stark, A. & Lohn, A. F. (1989). The use of verbalization in dance/movement therapy. *The Arts in Psychotherapy*, *16*(2), 105-113.

The authors propose that sound and speech positively influence the therapeutic process in dance/movement therapy. The literature reviewed includes the use of verbalization and vocalization in verbal psychotherapy and in dance/movement therapy. The authors offer two major categories of verbalization use in clinical work that enhance the integrating effect of dance/movement therapy. These categories include: a stimulus for body action, differentiation of self, recognition and expression of feelings, to aid in clarifying and providing insight into the personal content of the material in order to facilitate self-understanding.

107   Thom, R. A. (1975, December). Dance therapy: A different bouquet. *Dance Magazine*, p. 77.

This article offers a general picture of the profession of dance/movement therapy. The author focuses on observations for those considering a career in the field. The history of dance/movement therapy is traced. Populations with which dance/movement therapists work are outlined. A discussion of dance and postgraduate training for the therapist is presented. The American Dance Therapy Association is described in terms of goals and membership.

108   Wethered, A. (1973). *Movement and drama in therapy: The therapeutic use of movement, drama and music*. Boston, MA: Plays, Inc.

This book has been written to broaden the reader's understanding of both movement and therapeutic process. One section is focused exclusively on movement and therapy. Discussion includes: the principles of movement (e.g. Laban's effort qualities), movement work with patients, developing therapeutic themes and specific techniques and ways of using movement as therapy.

109   Whitehouse, M. (1977). The transference and dance therapy. <u>American Journal of Dance Therapy</u>, <u>1</u>(1), 3-7.

The author explores transference and projection from a Jungian perspective, beginning by examining the differences between Freud's and Jung's concepts of transference and projective identification. Citing case examples, the author illustrates the concepts of projection and transference, how they are different and how they are dealt with by the dance/movement therapist. Dance/movement therapy and psychoanalysis are contrasted, and the author states that the use of touch in dance/movement therapy is the intervention that sets it apart from analysis. Finally, the author compares trust in the therapeutic relationship and transference to enhance clarity in the sessions.

110   Whitehouse, M. (1970). Reflections on metamorphosis. <u>Impulse</u>, (Suppl.), 62-64.

The author traces her process of changing from dancer to therapist, from teaching dance class to enabling aliveness and expression. The discussion considers the differences between class and therapy, individual and group, and the conflict between technique and improvisation.

111   Willis, C. (1987). Legal and ethical issues of touch in dance/movement therapy. <u>American Journal of Dance Therapy</u>, <u>10</u>, 41-53.

The author describes the use of touch in dance/movement therapy followed by a discussion on the legal and ethical implications of touch between therapist and client, citing relevant cases. The author includes a "model for informed consent for touch in dance/movement therapy."

112   Woody, R. (1958). <u>Young dancer's career book</u>. New York: E. P. Dutton.

A chapter in this book contains information about dance/movement therapy as a career for the would be dancer who wants to be employed in the helping professions. The author gives basic rationale for the field by focusing on the populations potentially aided by dance/movement therapy. Quotes from various sources describing the work and its benefits are included.

113   Wooten, B. J. (1959). Movement therapy in England. *Journal of Health, Physical Education and Recreation*, *30*(6), 75-76.

The author considers the responses of British dance/movement therapists, psychiatrists and administrators to a questionnaire investigating England's field of dance/movement therapy. Common responses to the inquiry are discussed. These answers focus on exploring movement analysis in terms of diagnosis as a basis for treatment.

114   *Workshop on dance therapy: It's research potentials*. (1968). New York: Postgraduate Center for Mental Health.

The American Dance Therapy Association, Committee on Research in Dance and the Postgraduate Center for Mental Health joined together for this conference with the intent that persons in the fields of dance and psychotherapy gather to exchange ideas, with particular emphasis on more collaboration among the fields in research. A panel discussion and analysis of a group dance/movement therapy session led by Sharon Chaiklin and a videotaped individual dance/movement and verbal therapy session led by Mary Whitehouse is included.

CONFERENCE PROCEEDINGS AND MONOGRAPHS

115   American Dance Therapy Association. (1968). *Proceedings of the 3rd Annual Conference of the American Dance Therapy Association*. Columbia, MD: American Dance Therapy Association.

The topics explored at conference include: movement and personality, movement as human expression and artistic communication, the importance of science to the field's growth, linguistic-kinesic research, movement communication with children and the use of movement exercises for personal growth. The populations discussed are autism and geriatrics.

116   American Dance Therapy Association. (1969). *Proceedings of the 4th Annual Conference of the American Dance Therapy Association*. Columbia, MD: American Dance Therapy Association.

The papers presented cover a variety of theoretical subjects. Other forms of therapy are examined, including art, music, psychodrama and the encounter group. The material focusing exclusively on dance/movement therapy describe specific areas of interest within the field. These are: the similarities and differences between dance/movement therapy and other creative arts therapies, dance as a part of the life process, movement analysis as a therapeutic tool, dance/movement therapy in a community mental health center and the use of dynamics in inducing catharsis.

117   American Dance Therapy Association. (1970). *Proceedings of the 5th Annual Conference of the American Dance Therapy Association*. Columbia, MD: American Dance Therapy Association.

The content of the conference includes the following topics: Marian Chace, the role of the body in therapy, the impact of non-verbal communication, a study of the movement characteristics of hospitalized psychiatric patients, dance/movement therapy within a hospital framework, change as a therapeutic goal and dance in relation to culture. Dance/movement therapy with teenagers diagnosed with schizophrenia is described.

118   American Dance Therapy Association. (1972). <u>Proceedings of the 6th Annual Conference of the American Dance Therapy Association</u>. Columbia, MD: American Dance Therapy Association.

The content of this conference includes the following topics: the origins of dance, dance/movement therapy and total health, sensory awareness, theater games, Alexander technique, the use of video and film in dance/movement therapy, Hawkin's technique, and a composite description of work with individuals, families and groups. A cognitive development program for adults diagnosed with mental retardation who have a history of psychotic episodes is presented.

119   American Dance Therapy Association. (1973-74). <u>Writings on body movement and communication</u>. Monograph No. 3. Columbia, MD: American Dance Therapy Association.

The topics explored in the monograph include: the complimentary relationship between dance/movement therapy and occupational therapy, training for dance/movement therapists, group dance/movement therapy as a ritual process, long-term treatment in a psychiatric hospital and a theoretical framework for dance/movement therapy. The clinical populations include childhood disorders, mood disorders and schizophrenia.

120   Bernstein, P. (Ed.). (1974). Therapeutic process: Movement as integration. <u>Proceedings of the 9th Annual Conference of the American Dance Therapy Association</u>. Columbia, MD: American Dance Therapy Association.

This collection of papers includes three areas of study: theoretical considerations in dance/movement therapy, theory and it's application in dance/movement therapy, and research in nonverbal behavior and dance/movement therapy. Autism is discussed, with a description of the BRIAAC scale (Behavior Rating Instrument for Autistic and other Atypical Children), and developmental studies utilizing the BRIAAC scale.

121   Donelan, F. (Ed.). (1971). <u>Reprint of the Proceedings of the 2nd Annual Conference of the American Dance Therapy Association</u>. Columbia, MD: American Dance Therapy Association.

The contents of this conference include: a discussion of Hawkin's technique, dance/movement therapy's role in the therapeutic community, suggestions for diagnostic and therapeutic procedures in dance/movement therapy, an exploration of the definition of psychiatric health and sickness, and a method of organizing treatment teams in large psychiatric hospitals. Autism is also discussed.

122   Donelan, F. (1971). Writings on body movement and communication. <u>American Dance Therapy Association Monograph No. 1</u>. Columbia, MD: American Dance Therapy Association.

This monograph contains information in the following areas: the study of nonverbal interactions in the classroom, the development and execution of an experimental dance/movement therapy program, how the dance teacher is prepared to do therapy and a general discussion on psychotherapy. A description of dance/movement therapy with children and psychiatric day patients is included.

123   Donelan, F. (Ed.). (1972). Writings on body movement and communication. <u>American Dance Therapy Association Monograph No. 2</u>. Columbia, MD: American Dance Therapy Association.

This monograph includes the following topics: stimulating vocalization through movement, observing and interpreting movement, a study of the effort system of notation, body-dynamics in individual work, an inquiry into rhythm and the expression of emotion. The populations explored are childhood disorders, geriatrics and patients diagnosed with psychoses.

124   Govine, B. F. & Smallwood, J. C. (1973). What is dance therapy, really? <u>Proceedings of the 7th Annual Conference of the American Dance Therapy Association</u>. Columbia, MD: American Dance Therapy Association.

The materials presented at conference span a variety of topics and viewpoints. General areas discussed include: theoretical constructs and philosophies, related therapies, the training of dance/movement therapists, stimulating awareness through experiencing, movement description systems and the mind/body connection. Materials concerning autistic, adolescent and geriatric populations are provided.

125   Harris, J. (Ed.). (1978). Conference proceedings. <u>American Journal of Dance Therapy</u>, $\underline{2}$(2), 1-47.

A compilation of conference proceedings from the 1978 National Conference of the American Dance Therapy Association. The conference general theme was "theoretical and clinical issues." Information reflects a variety of concerns. The basic theoretical categories are integration of dance/movement therapy with other psychotherapies, the use of mythology, supervision, descriptions of theoretical frameworks (e.g., Jungian, psychoanalytic) and the fundamentals and expansion of the field. Clinical work with children, substance abuse, geriatric and couples populations is discussed.

126   Plunk-Burdick, D. M., Fulton, E. L. & Chaiklin, S. (Eds.). (1974). Dance therapist in dimension: Depth and diversity. <u>Proceedings of the 8th Annual Conference of the American Dance Therapy Association</u>. Columbia, MD: American Dance Therapy Association.

The conference proceedings cover a variety of subjects. The information presented can be categorized loosely into these headings: the experience of being a clinician, research, clinical work with various populations, historical information about the field and techniques or styles of practicing dance/movement therapy. The populations discussed are hospitalized adults, geriatric, adolescents, mental retardation and visual impairments.

SECTION II - CLINICAL PRACTICE
CHAPTER I
ADOLESCENT DISORDERS

American Dance Therapy Association. (1970). *Proceedings of the 5th Annual Conference of the American Dance Therapy Association.* Columbia, MD: American Dance Therapy Association.

+117

127   Berrol, C. F. (1981). A neurophysiologic approach to dance/movement therapy: Theory and practice. *American Journal of Dance Therapy,* 4(1), 72-84.

The author discusses dance/movement therapy from a neuropsychological perspective. The article comprises an exploration into theoretical constructs focusing on the models of Ayres and Kephart. With these frameworks as underpinning, the author describes the practical application of the neurophysiological approach to dance/movement therapy through a description of a short term program. Case examples of four teenage girls with multi-handicaps, including visual and hearing impairments, provide observations of the cross-model approach.

Bruno, C. (1981). Applications and implications of "structured analysis of movement sessions" for dance therapy. *The Arts in Psychotherapy,* 8(2), 127-133.

+17

Govine, B. F. & Smallwood, J. C. (1973). What is dance therapy, really? *Proceedings of the 7th Annual Conference of the American Dance Therapy Association.* Columbia, MD: American Dance Therapy Association.

+124

128   Johnson, D. R. & Eicher, V. (1990). The use of dramatic activities to facilitate dance therapy with adolescents. <u>The Arts in Psychotherapy</u>, <u>17</u>(2), 157-164.

The authors offer examples of nine dramatic activities for use in dance/movement therapy groups: chair game, adverbs, hat, areas, doors, environments, charades, Johnny Carson show and five-year projection. The purpose of these structures, as stated by the authors, is to engage adolescents in an atmosphere of trust and safety, and to reduce the fear of engulfment and the threat of intimacy that adolescents might feel during group dance/movement therapy.

Leatherbee, T. & Wood, S. (Eds.). (1985). <u>A primer for theoretical models and clinical work in dance/movement therapy</u>. Philadelphia, PA: Hahnemann University Medical College.

+63

Plunk-Burdick, D. M., Fulton, E. L. & Chaiklin, S. (Eds.). (1974). Dance therapist in dimension: Depth and diversity. <u>Proceedings of the 8th Annual Conference of the American Dance Therapy Association</u>. Columbia, MD: American Dance Therapy Association.

+126

129   Rogers, S. B. (1977). Contributions of dance therapy in a treatment program for retarded adolescents and adults. <u>Art Psychotherapy</u>, <u>4</u>(3-4), 195-197.

This study discusses the nonverbal communications of persons diagnosed with mental retardation. Using Laban's effort/shape system, nonverbal communication is assessed in terms of social relationship, complex movements and non-complex movements. The author concludes with the suggestion that dance/movement therapy acknowledges both emotional and cognitive functioning, pre-verbal and verbal communication, and concrete and abstract concepts.

Schmais, C. & Felber, D. J. (1977). Dance therapy process analysis: A method for observing and analyzing a dance therapy group. <u>American Journal of Dance Therapy</u>, <u>1</u>(2), 18-25.

+91

130 Toombs, M. R., Walker, J. & Bonney, H. L. (1965). Dance therapy for retarded adolescents. <u>Journal of Music Therapy</u>, <u>2</u>(4), 115-117.

The authors provide descriptions of the use of eurhythmics, creative dance and square dancing in dance/movement therapy with adolescent boys and girls diagnosed with mental retardation and with adaptive behavior levels II through V. Dance/movement therapy goals as stated by the authors are increased motor, sensory and social functioning.

CHAPTER 2
ANXIETY DISORDERS

131   Frost, M. C. S. (1984). Changing movement patterns and lifestyle in a blind, obsessive-compulsive. <u>American Journal of Dance Therapy</u>, <u>7</u>, 15-31.

A case study in which a dance/movement therapist works with a middle-aged male diagnosed with obsessive-compulsive personality disorder who also suffers hereditary retinitis pigmentosa. The author explores clients severely restricted range of movement and intense, focused calendar counting and hypothesizes that by widening client's range of motion, his mental "vision" might also widen. The results are not conclusive, however, there is a correlation between expanding his range of movement and decreasing calendar counting.

132   Gorden-Cohen, N. (1987). Vietnam and reality - the story of Mr. D. <u>American Journal of Dance Therapy</u>, <u>10</u>, 95-109.

A case study detailing short-term dance/movement therapy treatment with a Vietnam veteran diagnosed with post traumatic stress disorder on issues of anger, mistrust, intimacy and letting go. During group sessions, Mr. D. processes a dangerous and violent battle in which he witnesses his best friend's brutal murder. The author presents a therapeutic "aftermath," which acts as an epilogue to Mr. D.'s treatment. The author reflects upon his dance/movement therapy treatment upon discovering that he spent his tour of duty during the Vietnam war in Japan, and thus, could not have been in battle.

CHAPTER 3
CHILDHOOD DISORDERS

American Dance Therapy Association. (1968). <u>Proceedings of the 3rd Annual Conference of the American Dance Therapy Association</u>. Columbia, MD: American Dance Therapy Association.

+115

American Dance Therapy Association. (1972). <u>Proceedings of the 6th Annual Conference of the American Dance Therapy Association</u>. Columbia, MD: American Dance Therapy Association.

+118

American Dance Therapy Association. (1973-74). <u>Writings on body movement and communication</u>. Monograph No. 3. Columbia, MD: American Dance Therapy Association.

+119

Bernstein, P. (Ed.). (1974). Therapeutic process: Movement as integration. <u>Proceedings of the 9th Annual Conference of the American Dance Therapy Association</u>. Columbia, MD: American Dance Therapy Association.

+120

Berrol, C. F. (1981). A neurophysiologic approach to dance/movement therapy: Theory and practice. <u>American Journal of Dance Therapy</u>, <u>4</u>(1), 72-84.

+127

133 Berrol, C. F. (1989). A view from Israel: Dance/movement and the creative arts therapies in special education. <u>The Arts in Psychotherapy</u>, <u>16</u>(2), 81-90.

The author explores the use of the creative arts therapies at special schools in Israel, offering observations about programs in Jerusalem, Tel

Aviv, Ra'anana and Haifa. The training of creative arts therapists at four post-baccalaureate programs in Israel is outlined. They include: Haifa University, Levinsky College School of Music Education and Lesley College - all which offer dance/movement therapy degrees - and David Yellin Teachers College, which offers a diploma in music therapy. The author also discusses the historical basis of dance and music in Judaism, the history of arts in the United States, the Compulsory Education Law in Israel and the Education for All Handicapped Children's Act (PL 94-142) in the United States.

134   Berrol, C. F. (1987). <u>Israel: Dance/movement therapy and the creative arts therapies in special education</u>. New York: World Rehabilitation Fund, National Institute of Disability and Rehabilitation Research, United States Department of Education.

In this document, dance/movement therapy as it is used in Israel with children is explored. The author investigates Israel's education system and creative arts therapies. Observations of several visits to sites where dance/movement therapy is being used are offered. A discussion includes the historical basis for dance in Judaism, the history of the arts in the United States, and special education with creative arts therapies in the United States. The author closes with a discussion of the future of creative arts therapies in the United States, focusing on the National Coalition of Art Therapy Associations, and the American Dance Therapy Association's Project Focus, a long-range employment and promotion program for special education and medical rehabilitation.

135   Berrol, C. (1984). The effects of two movement therapy approaches on selected academic, physical and socio-behavioral measures of first grade children with learning and perceptual motor problems. <u>American Journal of Dance Therapy</u>, <u>7</u>, 32-48.

68 students, all of whom scored lower than the 25th percentile in academic achievement scores and who displayed poor socio-behavioral adjustment and

motor performance, were randomly assigned to either dance/movement therapy, sensory integration activities or a control group. Pre and post testing using the Children's Checking Test and the Connors Teacher Rating Scale measured the following behavioral attributes: balance and posture, body image, praxis, visual form perception, hyperactivity and sensory discrimination. Although results indicate trends favoring one or both of the experimental groups, the scores were not statistically significant.

136 Canino, L. (1964, October). The world opens. Dance Magazine, pp. 46-47.

An early article which offers dance/movement therapy techniques for children with physical handicaps who are confined to bed or live with external apparatii restricting their mobility. The author describes sessions using props (e.g., scarves, elastic) for tactile stimulation and motor control, rhythm, imagery and storytelling in developing themes for the sessions.

137 Cole, I. L. (1982). Movement negotiations with an autistic child. The Arts in Psychotherapy, 9(1), 49-53.

This author describes dance/movement therapy with a child diagnosed with autism. The author states the therapist's needs with the client: to help, not harm the client by supporting and caring for him, and to not be physically hurt or uncomfortable. The author also describes what he suspects are the child's needs: to be allowed choices in his activities, to be supported by the therapist in his choices, and to receive affection-approval on a body level from the therapist. The article illustrates how the interrelationship between the needs of the therapist and the client enhance the therapeutic process and help move it forward.

Costonis, M. (Ed.). (1978). Therapy in Motion. Urbana-Champaign, IL: University of Illinois Press.

+30

138   Couper, J. L. (1981). Dance therapy: Effects of motor performance of children with learning disabilities. *Physical Therapy*, *61*(1), 23-26.

An experiment in which the effect of dance/movement therapy as facilitator for vestibular stimulation and play activities in a sensory integrative therapy program is measured on the motor performance of children diagnosed with learning disabilities. Two groups of five children experienced either dance/movement therapy or sensory integrative therapy during a four week treatment period. Pretests and posttests on motor performance are given. The results show improved motor performance in both groups, with slightly higher gains in the dance/movement therapy group. This indicates that dance/movement therapy could serve as a vestibular stimulation activity comparable to the typical play activities in a sensory integrative therapy program.

Donelan, F. (Ed.) (1971). *Reprint of the Proceedings of the 2nd Annual Conference of the American Dance Therapy Association*. Columbia, MD: American Dance Therapy Association.

+121

Donelan, F. (Ed.). (1971). Writings on body movement and communication. *American Dance Therapy Association Monograph No. 1*. Columbia, MD: American Dance Therapy Association.

+122

Donelan, F. (Ed.). (1972). Writings on body movement and communication. *American Dance Therapy Association Monograph No. 2*. Columbia, MD: American Dance Therapy Association.

+123

139 Duggan, D. (1978). Goals and methods in dance therapy with severely multi-handicapped children. <u>American Journal of Dance Therapy</u>, <u>2</u>(1), 31-34.

 The author reviews the use of dance/movement therapy for children diagnosed with autism, cerebral palsy and mental retardation. Through the use of play, tactile and kinesthetic stimulation, props, and eye and body contact with the therapist in dance/movement therapy, the author hypothesizes growth in the areas of body image, emotional and cognitive development.

 Espenak, L. (1981). <u>Dance therapy: Theory and application</u>. Springfield, IL: Thomas.

 +46

 Feder, E. & Feder, B. (1977). Dance Therapy. <u>Psychology Today</u>, <u>10</u>(9), 76-80.

 +48

 Feder, E. & Feder, B. (1981). <u>The expressive arts therapies</u>. Englewood Cliffs, NJ: Prentice-Hall.

 +49

140 Franklin, S. (1979). Movement therapy and selected measures of body image in the trainable mentally retarded. <u>American Journal of Dance Therapy</u>, <u>3</u>(1), 43-50.

 In this pilot study, an experiment is performed to measure effects of dance/movement therapy on body image of persons diagnosed with trainable mental retardation. An adaptive physical education group is used as the control group. The results show a significantly higher improvement in body image of the experimental group in comparison to the control group.

Goodill, S. & Leatherbee, T. (Eds.). (1984). <u>A primer for assessment and evaluation in dance/movement therapy</u>. Philadelphia, PA: Hahnemann University.

+51

Govine, B. F. & Smallwood, J. C. (1973). What is dance therapy, really? <u>Proceedings of the 7th Annual Conference of the American Dance Therapy Association</u>. Columbia, MD: American Dance Therapy Association.

+124

141   Gunning, S. V. & Holmes, H. (1973). Dance therapy with psychotic children: Definition and quantitative evaluation. <u>Archives of General Psychiatry</u>, <u>28</u>(5), 707-713.

The authors designed dance/movement therapy groups to facilitate motor efficiency and modify irregular and disordered body movements of children with autism and psychoses. The authors developed a scale from the study that evaluates dance/movement therapy with this population. The Volwiler Body Movement Analysis Scale (VBMA) was used to provide quantitative information for 19 aspects of body movement. In the study, 65 children experience dance/movement therapy for two years. The results are improved scores on the VBMA, suggesting increased normal behavior and positive effects of dance/movement therapy as part of the treatment program.

Hanna, J. L. (1988). <u>Dance and Stress</u>. New York: AMS Press.

+52

142   Kalish-Weiss, B. I. (1988). Born blind and visually handicapped infants: Movement psychotherapy and assessment. <u>The Arts in Psychotherapy</u>, <u>15</u>(2), 101-108.

The author creates a rationale for the use of dance/movement therapy for infants with visual impairments. Movement assessment uncovered needs

and disturbances in the following areas: body
movement, relationship, communication, mastery,
vocalization, sound receptiveness and
psychobiological development. Examples from
clinical work describe dance/movement therapy
interns working on facilitating change in these
categories.

Kaveler, S. & Riess, B. F. (1977). Dance
therapy. <u>Transnational Mental Health Research
Newsletter</u>, <u>19</u>(1), 2-5.

+57

Leatherbee, T. & Wood, S. (Eds.). (1985). <u>A
primer for theoretical models and clinical work
in dance/movement therapy</u>. Philadelphia, PA:
Hahnemann University Medical College.

+63

143 Leventhal, M. B. (1980). Dance therapy. <u>Journal
of Physical Education and Recreation</u>, <u>51</u>(7),
33-35.

An exploration of the use of dance/movement
therapy with children with emotional disturbances
and learning disabilities. The author describes
some characteristics of these populations as well
as the therapist-child relationship. A model is
suggested as a guideline for therapeutic process.

144 Leventhal, M. B. (Ed.). (1980). <u>Movement and
growth: Dance therapy for the special child</u>.
New York: New York University Press.

This book provides a collection of topics shared
at a symposium honoring UNICEF's International
Year of the Child. Hosted by the graduate dance
therapy program at New York University, the
symposium presents theories, research, and methods
in dance/movement therapy. The book is divided
into three sections: theoretical considerations,
methods and assessments. The following topics are
presented: dance/movement therapy with the
special child, an introduction to
psychoanalytically-oriented dance/movement
therapy, a program for ego development with case

studies of children with emotional disturbances, methods in dance/movement therapy for children with learning disabilities, severe multi-handicaps, autism, non-verbal assessment of family systems and a brief description of the Behavior Rating Instrument for Autistic and Other Atypical Children (BRIAAC).

Levy, F. J. (1988). <u>Dance/movement therapy: A healing art</u>. Reston, VA: American Alliance for Health, Physical Education, Recreation and Dance.

+65

145 Liljenquist, J. (1984). <u>Dance/movement therapy in pediatrics</u>. Fairfax Co., VA: Agency for Cinema-Cartography.

The author presents dance/movement therapy for use with stressors children incur while hospitalized for physical illness. Working within a developmental framework, the author explores attachment, body ego integrity, defense mechanisms and children's reactions to stress during a hospital stay. Dance/movement therapy interventions offered include: creative games, play, and art activities to enhance the therapeutic relationship and to facilitate mastery, control and reinforcement of body image.

Mason, K. C. (Ed.). (1974). Dance therapy. <u>Focus on Dance VII</u>, 72. Washington, D.C.: American Alliance for Health, Physical Education and Recreation.

+68

Plunk-Burdick, D. M., Fulton, E. L. & Chaiklin, S. (Eds.). (1974). Dance therapist in dimension: Depth and diversity. <u>Proceedings of the 8th Annual Conference of the American Dance Therapy Association</u>. Columbia, MD: American Dance Therapy Association.

+126

146   Rakusin, A. (1990). A dance/movement therapy model incorporating movement education concepts for emotionally disturbed children. <u>The Arts in Psychotherapy</u>, <u>17</u>(1), 55-67.

The author explores the integration of movement education and dance/movement therapy. A model is suggested for combining the two in a clinical setting. The model is divided into six phases: welcome, warmup, thematic material, free movement, and relaxation and closure. Examples for movement education and dance/movement therapy interventions are woven into case material presented. The author includes basic outline for model in the appendix.

147   Razy, V. (1961). Value of dance and percussion in the treatment of emotionally disturbed children. <u>Social Casework</u>, <u>42</u>, 501-505.

The author suggests the use of percussion combined with dance to create useful adjunct therapy for children diagnosed with emotional disturbances. Two case illustrations are given from group dance and percussion therapy sessions.

148   Schmais, C. & Orleans, F. (1981). Dance/movement therapy with the MBD child. In R. Ochroch (Ed.), <u>The diagnosis and treatment of minimal brain dysfunction in children: A clinical approach</u> (pp. 166-179). New York: Human Sciences Press.

The dynamics, motivations, and aspirations of the child with minimal brain dysfunction are the focus of the authors' dance/movement therapy work with this population. Therapeutic issues of body awareness, spatial orientation, balance, eye-hand and eye-foot coordination, and arhythmicity are explored in dance/movement therapy facilitating work with the social, cognitive and motor deficits in the child with minimal brain dysfunction. The authors include three clinical vignettes illustrating dance/movement therapy interventions of mirroring, props, rhythm, folk dancing, and creative activities, while watching how the child performs the action through Laban's concepts of flow, time, force and space.

149   Schmerling, J. & Kerins, M. R. (1987). Stimulating communication in an elective mute: Collaborative interventions. <u>American Journal of Dance Therapy</u>, <u>10</u>, 27-40.

A case study in which dance/movement and speech/language therapists collaborate in working with a child diagnosed with elective mutism.

150   Schul, J. (1983). Exceptional children dancing: How special students gain ability and confidence through dance therapy. <u>Design for the Arts in Education</u>, <u>84</u>, 32-35.

This article outlines the author's work with the Very Special Creative Dance Program in Louisiana. Working with elementary age children with hearing impairments, emotional disturbances, learning disabilities, mental retardation and physical handicaps, the author explores issues of trust, expression of emotion and self esteem. The therapeutic interventions with the children include the use of drawings, stories, range of movement exercises and props to facilitate dance/movement therapy goals.

151   Shennum, W. A. (1987). Expressive activity therapy in residential treatment: Effects on children's behaviors in the treatment milieu. <u>Child and Youth Care Quarterly</u>, <u>16</u>(2), 81-90.

The hypothesis is suggested that expressive therapies (e.g., art, dance, movement) when used in milieu treatment program will decrease emotional unresponsiveness and acting out. 45 inpatient children diagnosed with emotional and behavior disturbances participated as subjects. The procedure presented three levels of participation: no expressive therapy, one hour per week of expressive therapy, or two hours per week of expressive therapy. The results show a positive effect.

Siegel, E. V. (1984). <u>Dance/movement therapy: Mirror of ourselves: The psychoanalytic approach</u>. New York: Human Sciences Press.

+98

152   Siegel, E. V. (1973). Movement therapy with autistic children. <u>Psychoanalytic Review</u>, <u>60</u>, 141-149.

A case study in which the author describes her work with four children diagnosed with schizophrenia and autism during nine months of dance/movement therapy sessions. The therapeutic goals include increased body awareness and sense of self. The author describes change as occurring on a physical (e.g., extinction of toe walking), social (e.g., the ability to join in movement tasks together), and self awareness (e.g., identifying body parts).

153   Siegel, E. V. & Blau, B. (1978). Breathing together: A preliminary investigation of an involuntary reflex as adaptation. <u>American Journal of Dance Therapy</u>, <u>2</u>(1), 35-42.

The authors work within developmental and psychoanalytic frames of reference to investigate the respiration patterns of children with psychotic diagnoses. Dance/movement therapy interventions using breathing to facilitate physiological and psychological development are explored. The article includes a study measuring the breathing patterns of 38 psychotic children. Forced Vital Capacity was measured between psychotic and normal children using the McKesson respirometer. Results indicate that psychotic children do exhibit diminished forced vital capacity. Suggestions for future research are presented by the authors.

154   Stephenson, S. (1959, March). To dance is to speak. <u>Dance Magazine</u>, pp. 56-57, 88-89.

An early article in which dance is used therapeutically with pre-school children with speech difficulties. A six-week intensive speech clinic is described with dance/movement therapy as the focus. Goals for the children are physical, social and psychological. The author provides four fundamentals that the dance/movement therapist must always consider. These are: the use of basic movement principles in an improvisational setting, the creation of new ways of moving, the encouragement for the children to find their own way of moving, and maintenance of a personal connection with the work and the children.

155 Weisbrod, J. (1972). Shaping a body image through movement therapy. Music Educators Journal, 58(8), 66-69.

This article is divided into two sections: the first section is an introduction to children's movements, movement fundamentals (e.g., strength, endurance, locomotion, time) and dance/movement therapy, and the second section includes a description of dance/movement therapy with various childhood disorders. These populations include children with hearing impairments, visual impairments, brain injuries, mental retardation and emotional disturbances.

CHAPTER 4
EATING DISORDERS

156   Krueger, D. & Schofield, E. (1986). Dance/movement therapy of eating disordered patients: A model. *The Arts in Psychotherapy*, *13*(4), 323-331.

This article begins with a discussion of the psychodynamic aspects of eating disorders and the development of body image. The authors then describe a developmental approach and introduce dance/movement therapy as a theory. The article concludes with suggested dance/movement therapy techniques. These include: relaxation and centering, mirroring each other, facing the mirror, projective drawings and videotaping.

Levy, F. J. (1988). *Dance/movement therapy: A healing art*. Reston, VA: American Alliance for Health, Physical Education, Recreation and Dance.

+65

157   Stark, A., Aronow, S., & McGeehan, T. (1989). Dance/movement therapy with bulimic patients. In L. M. Hornyak & E. K. Baker (Eds.), *Experiential therapies for eating disorders* (pp. 121-143). New York: The Guilford Press.

The authors focus on the therapeutic process and the goals of dance/movement therapy with patients diagnosed with bulimia nervosa. Also explored is group work and the movement characteristics of patients with bulimia. The authors define six treatment issues with this population: developing trust, developing body awareness and a realistic body image, developing a clearer sense of self and body boundaries, encouraging autonomy and enhancing self esteem, and encouraging interpersonal relationships and authentic self expression.

158   Wise, S. K. (1981). Dance/movement therapy as treatment in obesity. <u>Obesity and Metabolism</u>, <u>1</u>(1), 54-56.

The author introduces dance/movement therapy as an effective treatment for patients who are obese. The suggestion is made that because dance/movement therapy is an organic and authentic movement form from the patient's own repertoire, it is therefore a non-threatening form of therapy. Dance/movement therapy is recommended as a preferred form of treatment for those patients who use overeating, who are depressed, who are suppressing emotion, who have poor stress management skills, or who are experiencing recurrent emotional themes. The author suggests researching and documenting work with this population.

159   Wise, S. K. (1981). Dance therapy: Use of imagery for food awareness. <u>Obesity and Metabolism</u>, <u>1</u>(2), 96-104.

Movement and relaxation are presented as ways to stimulate Jung's principle of active imagination (e.g., stir images, fantasy, and memory) in order to relieve misuse of food. The author presents three methods of using dance/movement therapy with people suffering from eating disorders. These include: focusing on the body to discover physical or psychological hunger, using imagery to investigate emotional needs, and addressing somatic issues. Two case examples supply description and support for the author's ideas.

CHAPTER 5
FAMILY

American Dance Therapy Association. (1972). <u>Proceedings of the 6th Annual Conference of the American Dance Therapy Association</u>. Columbia, MD: American Dance Therapy Association.

+118

Bernstein, P. L. (Ed.). (1984). <u>Theoretical approaches in dance/movement therapy</u> (Vol II). Dubuque, IA: Kendall/Hunt.

Lewis, P. (Ed.). (1984). <u>Theoretical approaches in dance/movement therapy</u> (Vol. II). Dubuque, IA: Kendall/Hunt.

+9

160 Chambliss, L. (1982). Movement therapy and the shaping of the neuropsychological model. <u>American Journal of Dance Therapy</u>, <u>5</u>, 18-27.

The author explores the combination of dance/movement therapy, the concept of the truine brain and behavior, and the theory and technique of focusing as interrelated treatment for family therapy. A case study of a family in dance/movement therapy co-led by a dance/movement therapist and a psychiatrist is included.

Harris, J. (Ed.). (1978). Conference proceedings. <u>American Journal of Dance Therapy</u>, <u>2</u>(2), 1-47.

+125

Leatherbee, T. & Wood, S. (Eds.). (1985). <u>A primer for theoretical models and clinical work in dance/movement therapy</u>. Philadelphia, PA: Hahnemann University Medical College.

+63

161   Levick, M. & Dulicai, D. (1979). Interfaces of creativity: A mini-symposium. <u>Art Psychotherapy</u>, <u>6</u>(3), 150-153.

The authors explore the clinical implications of a dance/movement therapist and an art therapist in collaboration during family therapy. The authors offer insights into a session in which the patients were asked to draw pictures of their families and to role-play the members in the pictures. The authors discuss the conscious and unconscious content that emerges from the art work and the movement patterns, and conclude with a group discussion of the work of the session.

162   Murphy, J. M. (1979). The use of non-verbal and body movement techniques in working with families and infants. <u>Journal of Marital and Family Therapy</u>, <u>5</u>(4), 61-66.

The author presents an integration of dance/movement therapy theory and techniques with those of family therapy. The author describes the emergence of dysfunctional family patterns as arising in infants early developments. Examples of dysfunctional interactions and therapeutic interventions are provided.

CHAPTER 6
GERIATRIC

American Dance Therapy Association. (1968). <u>Proceedings of the 3rd Annual Conference of the American Dance Therapy Association</u>. Columbia, MD: American Dance Therapy Association.

+115

163   Caplow-Lindner, E. (1979). <u>Therapeutic dance/movement: Expressive activities for older adults</u>. New York: Human Sciences Press.

The author provides theoretical material and programs developed for group work with four segments of the elderly spectrum: the well aged, the physically limited, the severely handicapped, and the withdrawn and regressed. The author's premise is that the lives of the elderly can be enriched through dance/movement therapy.

Donelan, F. (Ed.). (1972). Writings on body movement and communication. <u>American Dance Therapy Association Monograph No. 2</u>. Columbia, MD: American Dance Therapy Association.

+123

164   Fersh, I. E. (1980). Dance/movement therapy: A holistic approach to working with the elderly. <u>American Journal of Dance Therapy</u>, <u>3</u>(2), 33-43.

Fersh, I. E. (1981). Dance/movement therapy: A holistic approach to working with the elderly. <u>Activities, Adaptation and Aging</u>, <u>2</u>(1), 21-30.

This article centers on the authors premise that dance/movement therapy maximizes life growth potential. The author presents an introduction to the aging process, suggests methods of dance/movement therapy (e.g. reflecting movement, assessing movement preferences, and enlarging the movement repertoire) and discusses special populations within the parameters of geriatrics.

165   Goldberg, W. G. & Fitzpatrick, J. J. (1980). Movement therapy with the aged. <u>Nursing Research</u>, <u>29</u>(6), 339-346.

The authors hypothesize that dance/movement therapy will positively effect geriatric patients by raising morale and self esteem, decreasing loneliness and agitation and improving attitudes towards aging. Subjects were drawn from a residential facility. The experimental group participated in six weeks of dance/movement therapy led by nurses. The results substantiate the hypotheses on all measures.

Goodill, S. & Leatherbee, T. (Eds.). (1984). <u>A primer for assessment and evaluation in dance/movement therapy</u>. Philadelphia, PA: Hahnemann University.

+51

Govine, B. F. & Smallwood, J. C. (1973). What is dance therapy, really? <u>Proceedings of the 7th Annual Conference of the American Dance Therapy Association</u>. Columbia, MD: American Dance Therapy Association.

+124

Hanna, J. L. (1988). <u>Dance and Stress</u>. New York: AMS Press.

+53

Harris, J. (Ed.). (1978). Conference proceedings. <u>American Journal of Dance Therapy</u>, <u>2</u>(2), 1-47.

+125

Leatherbee, T. & Wood, S. (Eds.). (1985). <u>A primer for theoretical models and clinical work in dance/movement therapy</u>. Philadelphia, PA: Hahnemann University Medical College.

+63

Levy, F. J. (1988). <u>Dance/movement therapy: A healing art</u>. Reston, VA: American Alliance for Health, Physical Education, Recreation and Dance.

+65

166 Lindner, E. C. (1982). Dance as a therapeutic intervention for the elderly. <u>Educational Gerontology</u>, <u>8</u>(2), 167-174.

The author suggests the use of dance/movement therapy as a primary intervention for the elderly. A discussion of therapeutic effects compose the bulk of the article. These effects include: increased self esteem and communication, enhanced reminiscence and socialization and improved organization and sense of wellness.

Mason, K. C. (Ed.). (1974). Dance therapy. <u>Focus on Dance VII</u>, 72. Washington, D.C.: American Alliance for Health, Physical Education and Recreation.

+68

167 Mason-Luckey, B. & Sandel, S. L. (1985). Intergenerational movement therapy: A leadership challenge. <u>The Arts in Psychotherapy</u>, <u>12</u>(4), 257-263.

The authors bring together inner-city elementary school children with residents of a long-term care residential facility for twelve movement and music sessions. Interventions include structures that engage both populations while facilitating spontaneous interaction, such as games that encourage fantasy and hope, the use of rhythm, development of rituals and chanting circle games. These dance/movement therapy processes evoke constructive relationships, vocalization, imagining, and sharing. The authors suggest that the children learn self control and develop self esteem, and that the elderly are revitalized by the shared experience.

Plunk-Burdick, D. M., Fulton, E. L. & Chaiklin, S. (Eds.). (1974). Dance therapist in dimension: Depth and diversity. <u>Proceedings of the 8th Annual Conference of the American Dance Therapy Association</u>. Columbia, MD: American Dance Therapy Association.

+126

168   Sandel, S. L. (1984). Creating and playing: Bridges for intergenerational communication. <u>Design for Arts in Education</u>, <u>86</u>, 32-35.

Project TOUCH brings together residents of a long-term care geriatric facility and inner-city school children, kindergarten through grade five. The author parallels issues of both populations as poorly developed verbal skills and low self esteem, and cites the challenge of the dance/movement therapist as bridging the generations with common therapeutic themes. The author uses rhythmic movement, song, clay and dramatic play as interventions and discusses the benefits of the program.

169   Sandel, S. L. (1978). Movement therapy with geriatrics in a convalescent home. <u>Hospital and Community Psychiatry</u>, <u>29</u>(11), 738-741.

The author discusses the process of creating a dance/movement therapy program for long-term geriatric patients in a convalescent home, including educating the staff about dance/movement therapy and establishing the culture of the groups. Issues of trust, touch, stimulating vocalization, socialization and communicating anger and despair in the group sessions are explored with a final note about changes in behavior, notably increased communication among the patients.

170   Sandel, S. L. (1978). Reminiscence in movement therapy with the aged. <u>Art Psychotherapy</u>, <u>5</u>(4), 217-221.

Reminiscence is recommended as an appropriate means for stimulating peer interaction, cognitive organization and increased self-esteem with geriatric populations. The author offers examples from group dance/movement therapy.

171 Sandel, S. L. (1979). Sexual issues in movement therapy with geriatric patients. American Journal of Dance Therapy, 3(1), 4-14.

The author illustrates use of dance/movement therapy in addressing sexuality and intimacy with geriatric patients. The common issues may include loneliness, fear of physical deterioration, anger, sexual frustration, desiring companionship and neediness. The article includes an individual case study as well as examples from group sessions.

172 Sandel, S. L. & Johnson, D. R. (1987). Waiting at the gate: Creativity and hope in the nursing home. New York: Haworth Press.

The authors illustrate the healing elements of movement and drama while structuring a therapeutic and growth enhancing community in a nursing facility. Clinical issues addressed are: reminiscence and exploring sexual issues in dance/movement therapy, expressive group therapy with severely confused patients, intergenerational dance/movement therapy and therapeutic rituals in the nursing home.

173 Unger, A. (1985). Movement therapy for the geriatric population. Clinical Gerontologist, 3(3), 46-47.

The author provides clinical comments on her work with the elderly. Dance/movement therapy is suggested as means of fulfilling patients intrinsic needs. These needs as defined by the author are to experience fulfillment, control, belonging, tolerance and to recognize the self as unique. The article presents the author's techniques with this population and describes the basic process of a group dance/movement therapy session.

CHAPTER 7
MOOD DISORDERS

American Dance Therapy Association. (1973-74). *Writings on body movement and communication*. Monograph No. 3. Columbia, MD: American Dance Therapy Association.

+119

174 Grodner, S., Braff, D., Janowsky, D. & Clopton, P. (1982). Efficacy of art/movement therapy in elevating mood. *The Arts in Psychotherapy*, *9*(3), 217-225.

Using an inpatient psychiatric setting, the authors test the hypothesis that after receiving combined art and dance/movement therapy, patients will perceive an elevation in mood and group interaction. Subjects include 45 patients diagnosed with schizophrenia, psychotic depression and depression, as well as ten normal staff members. Comparing the effects on a directed art/movement activity, a non-directed art activity and a no-treatment group, authors utilize McNair's The Profile of Mood Status (POMS) Scale and The Semantic Differential Scale for pre-treatment and post-treatment testing. Results indicated a significant improvement in mood over the course of treatment in the directed art/movement activity group.

175 Sandel, S. L. & Johnson, D. R. (1983). Structure and process of the nascent group: Dance therapy with chronic patients. *The Arts in Psychotherapy*, *10*(3), 131-140.

The authors present a case study of a nascent group. The course of the group development is organized into phases in terms of relatedness. These phases are categorized as: high hopes or social facade, the struggle for relatedness or collapse and gestation, and termination or disillusion. Therapist countertransference is also addressed.

CHAPTER 8
NEUROSES

Bernstein, P. L. (Ed.). (1984). <u>Theoretical approaches in dance/movement therapy</u> (Vol II). Dubuque, IA: Kendall/Hunt.

Lewis, P. (Ed.). (1984). <u>Theoretical approaches in dance/movement therapy</u> (Vol. II). Dubuque, IA: Kendall/Hunt.

+9

Chambliss, L. (1982). Movement therapy and the shaping of the neuropsychological model. <u>American Journal of Dance Therapy</u>, <u>5</u>, 18-27.

+160

176   Cheney, G. (1970). "It is a gift." <u>Impulse</u>, (Suppl.), 65-68.

The author uses her own experience in dance/movement therapy as a client to describe the process of change in "movement in depth," Mary Whitehouse's form of dance/movement therapy. She then presents a scenario from her class in which she uses her new knowledge and changed self to allow her students an opportunity to express their emotions.

177   Cohen, B. M. (1983). Combined art and movement therapy group: Isomorphic responses. <u>The Arts in Psychotherapy</u>, <u>10</u>(4), 229-232.

The author recommends combined group sessions of art and dance/movement therapy as means to create isomorphic responses to increase therapeutic potential. Labans's effort categories are compared to drawing change categories. The author suggests this correlation: bound, direct, heavy, sudden with increased intensity, free, indirect, light, sustained with decreased intensity and increased flexibility, and idiosyncratic with increased organization.

Duggan, D. (1981). Dance therapy. In R. Corsini (Ed.), <u>Innovative Psychotherapies</u>, (pp. 229-240). New York: Wiley & Sons.

+44

Espenak, L. (1981). <u>Dance therapy: Theory and application</u>. Springfield, IL: Thomas.

+46

Evan, B. (1959, November). Therapeutic aspects of creative dance. <u>Dance Observer</u>, pp.?

Evan, B. (1967). <u>The child's world: It's relation to dance pedagogy</u>. New York: St. Marks Editions.

The author offers brief comments on dance/movement therapy in terms of types of clients, therapists, teachers and the psychotherapeutic community. A discussion of the importance of knowing and working with an awareness of physical and psychological limits and weaknesses of clients is presented. The clients are categorized as normal, normally disturbed, neurotic, psychotic and disabled. Suggestions for the would-be therapist are included.

Feder, E. & Feder, B. (1981). <u>The expressive arts therapies</u>. Englewood Cliffs, NJ: Prentice-Hall.

+50

Goodill, S. & Leatherbee, T. (Eds.). (1984). <u>A primer for assessment and evaluation in dance/movement therapy</u>. Philadelphia, PA: Hahnemann University.

+51

179 Greenberg, T. R. (1978). Two case studies - a dance therapy process. <u>Journal of Biological Experience</u>, <u>1</u>(1), 35-45.

Berlin, A. L. & Greenberg, T. R. (1980). <u>Move and be moved: A practical approach to movement with meaning</u>. Los Angeles, CA: Learning Through Movement.

This article presents two case studies of adult women as clients in dance/movement therapy. The author describes the process of change that the clients experience. Discussion of the similarities and differences between the two clients focuses on boundaries, experiencing, flexibility and the space between extremes.

Johnson, D. R., Sandel, S. L. & Eicher, V. (1983). Structural aspects of group leadership styles. <u>American Journal of Dance Therapy</u>, <u>6</u>, 17-31.

+56

Kaveler, S. & Riess, B. F. (1977). Dance therapy. <u>Transnational Mental Health Research Newsletter</u>, <u>19</u>(1), 2-5.

+57

Leatherbee, T. & Wood, S. (Eds.). (1985). <u>A primer for theoretical models and clinical work in dance/movement therapy</u>. Philadelphia, PA: Hahnemann University Medical College.

+63

180 Leste, A. & Rust, J. (1984). Effects of dance on anxiety. <u>Perceptual and Motor Skills</u>, 1984, <u>58</u>, 767-772.

Leste, A. & Rust, J. (1990). Effects of dance on anxiety. <u>American Journal of Dance Therapy</u>, <u>12</u>(1), 19-25.

The authors conduct an experiment in dance/movement therapy to measure the effect of dance on anxiety while controlling for physical exercise and music. Subjects include 114 college age students who completed pretest and posttest questionnaires, and results were measured using the Spielberger State-Trait Anxiety Inventory. The results indicate that dance, unlike any of the control activities, significantly reduces anxiety.

Levy, F. J. (1988). <u>Dance/movement therapy: A healing art</u>. Reston, VA: American Alliance for Health, Physical Education, Recreation and Dance.

+65

181 Meyer, S. (1985). Women and conflict in dance therapy. <u>Women and Therapy</u>, <u>4</u>(1), 3-17.

The author describes her understanding of the therapeutic relationship, and conflict as it is experienced and expressed by women. The article is divided into sections discussing initial experiences in therapy, the process of working through conflicts and termination. Clinical examples are given from the author's work as a dance/movement therapist.

North, M. <u>Personality assessment through movement</u>. Boston, MA: Plays, Inc.

+74

Smallwood, J. Dance therapy and the transcendent function. <u>American Journal of Dance Therapy</u>, <u>2</u>(1), 16-23.

+103

CHAPTER 9
PERSONALITY DISORDERS

Bruno, C. (1981). Applications and implications of "structured analysis of movement sessions" for dance therapy. <u>The Arts in Psychotherapy</u>, <u>8</u>(2), 127-133.

+17

Dosamantes-Alperson, E. (1987). Transference and countertransference issues in movement psychotherapy. <u>The Arts in Psychotherapy</u>, <u>14</u>(3), 209-214.

+41

Feder, E. & Feder, B. (1977). Dance Therapy. <u>Psychology Today</u>, <u>10</u>(9), 76-80.

+48

Johnson, D. R., Sandel, S. L. & Eicher, V. (1983). Structural aspects of group leadership styles. <u>American Journal of Dance Therapy</u>, <u>6</u>, 17-31.

+56

182 Kalish-Weiss, B. I. (1982). Attachment and separation: Major themes in movement therapy with adults. <u>The Arts in Psychotherapy</u>, <u>9</u>(4), 249-257.

The author suggests the use of a developmental framework in dance/movement therapy. Individual case studies describe clients working through the attachment and separation process. Stages of development are paralleled to experiences within the therapy sessions.

183   Naess, J. (1982). A developmental approach to the interactive process in dance/movement therapy. *American Journal of Dance Therapy*, *5*, 43-55.

Based on the developmental theories of Margaret Mahler, the author presents case studies of individual and group work with two young women diagnosed with borderline personality disorder and schizophrenia, chronic, undifferentiated type. The author applies movement response patterns and non-verbal cues to the developmental framework, and explores the following factors: degree of ego boundary, use of space, passivity or activity, imitation, touch, friction and compliance.

184   Ragan, C. & Seides, M. (1990). The synthetic use of movement and verbal psychoanalytic psychotherapies. In A. L. S. Silver & M. B. Cantor (Eds.), *Psychoanalysis and severe emotional illness* (pp. 115-130). New York: Guilford Press.

A case study in which the authors work from psychoanalytic paradigm. A dance/movement therapist and psychiatrist share primary therapy with female inpatient diagnosed with borderline personality disorder and epilepsy. The authors use dance/movement therapy to facilitate and enhance movement transferences, thus accessing psychosomatic potential space and increasing transferences in the verbal psychotherapy.

Robbins, A. (1980). *Expressive therapy: A creative arts approach to depth-oriented treatment*. New York: Human Sciences Press.

+80

Siegel, E. V. (1984). *Dance/movement therapy: Mirror of ourselves: The psychoanalytic approach*. New York: Human Sciences Press.

+98

CHAPTER 10
PHYSICAL AND SEXUAL ABUSE

Dosamantes-Alperson, E. (1987). Transference and countertransference issues in movement psychotherapy. The Arts in Psychotherapy, 14(3), 209-214.

+41

185   Goodill, S. (1987). Dance/movement therapy with abused children. The Arts in Psychotherapy, 14(1), 59-68.

The author suggests dance/movement therapy as a vehicle for neglected children who have been physically and sexually abused. Clinical vignettes demonstrate the modality's usefulness in facilitating trust, exploring feelings, acknowledging past traumas, creating a new identity and changing behavior patterns.

Levy, F. J. (1988). Dance/movement therapy: A healing art. Reston, VA: American Alliance for Health, Physical Education, Recreation and Dance.

+65

186   Weltman, M. (1986). Movement therapy with children who have been sexually abused. American Journal of Dance Therapy, 9, 47-66.

The author reviews literature on sexual abuse and presents dance/movement therapy as an effective modality for diagnosing and treating children who have been sexually abused. A case study illustrates clients working through the traumatic effects of the abuse. The effects are centered in four areas, including relationship patterns, self esteem, sexual identity and body image.

CHAPTER 11
SCHIZOPHRENIA

American Dance Therapy Association. (1973-74). <u>Writings on body movement and communication</u>. Monograph No. 3. Columbia, MD: American Dance Therapy Association.

+119

American Dance Therapy Association. (1970). <u>Proceedings of the 5th Annual Conference of the American Dance Therapy Association</u>. Columbia, MD: American Dance Therapy Association.

+117

Bainbridge, G., Duddington, A. E., Collingdon, M. & Gardner, C. E. (1953). Dance-mime: A contribution to treatment in psychiatry. <u>Journal of Mental Science</u>, <u>99</u>, 308-314.

+4

Bruno, C. (1981). Applications and implications of "structured analysis of movement sessions" for dance therapy. <u>The Arts in Psychotherapy</u>, <u>8</u>(2), 127-133.

+17

Christup, H. J. (1962). The effect of dance therapy on the concept of body image. <u>Psychiatric Quarterly Supplement</u>, <u>36</u>(1), 296-303.

The use of projective drawing tests administered before and after dance/movement therapy sessions measure dance/movement therapy's impact on the concept of body image with chronic hospitalized patients diagnosed with schizophrenia. The results indicate that dance/movement therapy produced a positive change in body image with women more than with men and with participants who were more active in the group session.

Cohen, B. M. (1984). Combined art and movement therapy group: Isomorphic responses. <u>The Arts in Psychotherapy</u>, <u>10</u>(4), 229-232.

+177

Costonis, M. (Ed.). (1978). <u>Therapy in Motion</u>. Urbana-Champaign, IL: University of Illinois Press.

+30

188 Dondinger, R. A. & Trop, J. L. (1979). Combined physical and psychiatric disabilities: A case study in movement therapy. <u>American Journal of Dance Therapy</u>, <u>3</u>(1), 15-19.

A case study in which the authors describe the therapeutic process, goals, and achievements of a patient with combined visual impairment due to self-mutilation and a psychiatric disorder that includes delusions and auditory hallucinations. Dance/movement therapy goals include facilitating a sense of control, maintaining a clear sense of internal boundaries and expansion of the patient's movement repertoire. The author concludes with reflections about how dance/movement therapy provided an integral structure for this patient's treatment and eventual growth during recovery.

Dosamantes-Alperson, E. (1974). The creation of meaning through body movement. In A. I. Rabin (Ed.), <u>Clinical psychology: Issues of the seventies</u>. (pp. 156-165). E. Lansing, MI: Michigan State University Press.

+38

189 Ehrhardt, B. T., Hearn, M. B. & Novak, C. (1989). Outpatient clients attitudes towards healing processes in dance therapy. <u>American Journal of Dance Therapy</u>, <u>11</u>(1), 39-60.

A three part experiment including an interview, a revised interview and a validation study to measure chronic psychiatric patients' attitudes towards healing processes in dance/movement therapy. Measured on videotape were eight healing processes as developed by Schmais: rhythm, cohesion, vitalization, synchrony, expression, exercise, music and relaxation. Patients viewed the videotape and ranked the segment they liked the most, vitalization; the second most, exercise; and the least, music. The authors conclude that patients are aware of, have attitudes about, and can rank healing processes in order of preference.

Espenak, L. (1981). <u>Dance therapy: Theory and application</u>. Springfield, IL: Thomas.

+46

Evans, B. (1959, November). Therapeutic aspects of creative dance. <u>Dance Observer</u>, pp. _____.

Evans, B. (1967). <u>The child's world: It's relation to dance pedagogy</u>. New York: St. Marks Editions.

+178

Feder, E. & Feder, B. (1981). <u>The expressive arts therapies</u>. Englewood Cliffs, NJ: Prentice-Hall.

+50

Goodill, S. & Leatherbee, T. (Eds.). (1984). <u>A primer for assessment and evaluation in dance/movement therapy</u>. Philadelphia, PA: Hahnemann University.

+51

Grodner, S., Braff, D., Janowsky, D. & Clopton, P. (1982). Efficacy of art/movement therapy in elevating mood. <u>The Arts in Psychotherapy</u>, <u>9</u>(3), 217-225.

+174

Harris, J. (Ed.). (1978). Conference proceedings. <u>American Journal of Dance Therapy</u>, <u>2</u>(2), 1-47.

+125

Johnson, D. R., Sandel, S. L. & Eicher, V. (1983). Structural aspects of group leadership styles. <u>American Journal of Dance Therapy</u>, <u>6</u>, 17-31.

+56

Kalish-Weiss, B. I. (1982). Attachment and separation: Major themes in movement therapy with adults. <u>The Arts in Psychotherapy</u>, <u>9</u>(4), 249-257.

+182

Kaveler, S. & Riess, B. F. (1977). Dance therapy. <u>Transnational Mental Health Research Newsletter</u>, <u>19</u>(1), 2-5.

+57

Lavender, J. (1977). Moving toward meaning. <u>Psychotherapy: Theory, Research and Practice</u>, <u>14</u>(2), 123-133.

In this case study, the author recounts individual, long term treatment with a male inpatient diagnosed with schizophrenia, chronic, undifferentiated type. The author offers in-depth notes from dance/movement therapy sessions over a two year period. The author concludes with reflections on her growth as a young therapist, the therapist/patient relationship, and the role that dance as an art plays in the development of the therapeutic process.

Levy, F. J. (1988). <u>Dance/movement therapy: A healing art</u>. Reston, VA: American Alliance for Health, Physical Education, Recreation and Dance.

+65

May, R. (1941). Modern dancing as a therapy for the mentally ill. <u>Occupational Therapy and Rehabilitation</u>, <u>20</u>, 101-106.

+69

McCarthy, H. (1973). The use of the draw-a-person test to evaluate a dance therapy program. <u>Journal of Music Therapy</u>, <u>10</u>(3), 141-155.

+70

Naess, J. (1982). A developmental approach to the interactive process in dance/movement therapy. <u>American Journal of Dance Therapy</u>, <u>5</u>, 43-55.

+183

Rosen, E. (1974). <u>Dance in psychotherapy</u>. New York: Dance Horizons.

+81

Rosen, E. (1954). Dance therapy for the mentally ill. <u>Teacher's College Record</u>, <u>55</u>, 215-222.

In exploration of dance as therapy, the author questions how dance/movement therapy will help patients. Two groups are formed from patients diagnosed with psychoses from an inpatient setting. Both receive dance/movement therapy sessions. As a result of these experiences, the author summarizes how patients use dance to express themselves. Six categories are presented: withdrawn reaction, defensive over-reaction, aggressive reaction, exhibitionistic reaction, intellectual-defense reaction and voyeuristic identification reaction. The author concludes that dance/movement therapy provides a context where emotionally charged material can be communicated in a socially appropriate way.

192   Rosenberg, S. (1968). Dance therapy - a means of communication. <u>Psychiatric Communications</u>, <u>10</u>(1), 19-24.

The author discusses the use of dance for the mentally ill and offers an historical perspective through the work of pioneer Marian Chace. Chace's background as a dance teacher and her work as a dance/movement therapist at St. Elizabeths Hospital in Washington, D.C. is outlined. The author includes an illustration of a dance/movement therapy session containing a word for word dialogue between the therapist and the patients before and during the session. The author then discusses this session in terms of principles and dynamics of dance/movement therapy, and explores the concepts of kinesthetic empathy and rhythm. The author concludes with a discussion of the physical spaces in which dance/movement therapy can occur.

193   Sandel, S. L. (1980). Countertransference stress in the treatment of schizophrenic patients. <u>American Journal of Dance Therapy</u>, <u>3</u>(2), 20-32.

The therapist's internal experience and countertransference while working with patients diagnosed with schizophrenia is examined. Specific aspects addressed include helplessness, intense emotional involvement, passivity, the therapist's personal investment in movement and patients' sensitivity to the therapist's unconscious.

194   Sandel, S. L. (1980). Dance therapy in the psychiatric hospital. <u>Journal of the National Association of Private Psychiatric Hospitals</u>, <u>11</u>(2), 20-26.

The author begins with a brief history of dance/movement therapy and progresses to a discussion of dance/movement therapy as group and individual treatment with psychotic patients residing in a facility that emphasizes therapeutic community. Goals for this population as stated by the author are: developing body awareness and integration, increasing peer interaction, and expressing feelings in an appropriate and channeled way. The author also explores the patients's internalization of the norms and values of a group culture, and includes brief case illustrations of her work in group and individual dance/movement therapy.

195 Sandel, S. L. (1982). The process of individuation in dance/movement therapy with schizophrenic patients. *The Arts in Psychotherapy*, *9*, 11-18.

The author explores process of separation-individuation in dance/movement therapy with patients diagnosed with schizophrenia. The author describes the therapist's need to tolerate patient needs and own countertransference as paramount to promoting timely exploration of autonomy. Touch, sexuality and session structure are discussed in terms of both group and individual sessions.

Sandel, S. L. & Johnson, D. R. (1983). Structure and process of the nascent group: Dance therapy with chronic patients. *The Arts in Psychotherapy*, *10*(3), 131-140.

+175

Sandel, S. L. & Johnson, D. R. (1977). Structured analysis of group movement sessions: Preliminary research. *American Journal of Dance Therapy*, *1*(2), 32-36.

+84

196 Schoop, T. & Mitchell, P. (1974). *Won't you join the dance? A dancer's essay into the treatment of psychosis*. Palo Alto, CA: National Press.

The author describes the experience of becoming a dance/movement therapist including the conceptual material that is the basis of her style of treatment. The elements highlighted are breath, alignment, center, tension, rhythm, space, improvisation and formulation. Clinical examples of patients movements and interactions are used in combination with theoretical material to complete picture.

197 Skove, E. (1986). The psychosocial effects on the dance/movement therapist working with a schizophrenic population. *American Journal of Dance Therapy*, *9*, 67-82.

This pilot study examines the psychophysical effects of treating patients diagnosed with schizophrenia on dance/movement therapists. Therapists working with this population are interviewed. Results yield information on therapist background, interventions, experiences and preparatory and recuperative measures. Results also suggest that the effects of working with this population include weakened boundaries and depressed physical energy and emotions.

Siegel, E. V. (1984). *Dance/movement therapy: Mirror of ourselves: The psychoanalytic approach*. New York: Human Sciences Press.

+98

Siegel, E. V. (1973). Movement therapy with autistic children. *Psychoanalytic Review*, *60*, 141-149.

+152

198 Silberstein, S. (1987). Dance therapy and schizophrenia: A vision for the future. *The Arts in Psychotherapy*, *14*(2), 143-152.

The author begins this article by reviewing literature on schizophrenia. Based on this literature and an exploration of the behavioral and psychological etiology of schizophrenia, literature in psychoanalytic theory, Laban's effort/shape methods and the work of pioneers Chace and Schoop with patients with schizophrenia, the author provides a synthesis of the theories of dance/movement therapy and schizophrenia. A case vignette of the author's work with an elderly man with a diagnosis of mute schizophrenia, catatonic type is included. The author concludes with comments on the need for a strong theoretical framework in dance/movement therapy to contend with issues arising from patients diagnosed with schizophrenia.

199   Yula, B. (1984). Using creative movement to develop a potential space with the schizophrenic patient. *Pratt Institute Creative Art Therapy Review*, *5*, 12-16.

Attachment and object relations theories provide the framework for the author's work with a 59 year old female diagnosed with schizophrenia, chronic, undifferentiated type. Case illustration includes the patients' process of symbiosis and attachment through the beginning of separation. The author explores the concept of potential space while choosing a physical environment for treatment, and facilitating intrapsychic autonomy with the patient. Issues of transference and countertransference during the patients' struggle for autonomy, strength and mastery are also explored.

CHAPTER 12
SOMATIC DISORDERS

200   Bernstein, P. L. (1980). A mythological quest: Jungian movement therapy with the psychosomatic client. *American Journal of Dance Therapy*, *3*(2), 44-55.

The author offers case study of woman with rheumatoid arthritis to illustrate the strengths of Jungian dance/movement therapy for clients with psychosomatic diagnoses. The Jungian technique of active imagination combined with authentic movement in-depth are used by the author as means to uncover, communicate her client's unconscious material, as well as a tool for providing the direction of therapy.

Liljenquist, J. (1984). *Dance/movement therapy in pediatrics*. Fairfax Co., VA: Agency for Cinema-Cartography.

+145

Ragan, C. & Seides, M. (1990). The synthetic use of movement and verbal psychoanalytic psychotherapies. In A. L. S. Silver & M. B. Cantor (Eds.), *Psychoanalysis and severe emotional illness* (pp. 115-130). New York: Guilford Press.

+184

201   Seides, M. R. (1986). Dance/movement therapy as a modality in the treatment of the psychosocial complications of heart disease. *American Journal of Dance Therapy*, *9*, 83-101.

This article explores dance/movement therapy as treatment for psychosocial problems associated with heart disease. The author describes the coronary prone personality (e.g., excessively competitive, restless and aggressive). The coping skills arising from illness that may be effectively treated by dance/movement therapy are: denial, continuing to over-do, quitting or cardiac neurosis. The author presents therapeutic goals (e.g., creating realistic body image and externalizing thoughts and feelings). Case examples are given from group dance/movement therapy sessions and potential problems are suggested.

202 Silberman-Diehl, L. & Komisaruk, B. (1985). Treating psychogenic somatic disorders through body metaphor. *American Journal of Dance Therapy*, *8*, 37-45.

The authors focus on use of the body as a metaphor for experiencing, expressing and working through disorders. Case illustrations from dance/movement therapy sessions provide examples of clinical use of authors theories.

203 Westbrook, B. K. & McKibben, H. (1989). Dance/movement therapy with groups of outpatients with Parkinson's disease. *American Journal of Dance Therapy*, *11*(1), 27-38.

An experiment in which the authors hypothesize that dance/movement therapy is a more effective treatment modality on mood than exercise and movement initiation in patients with Parkinson's disease. Thirty-seven ambulatory Parkinsonian patients participated in twelve weeks of dance/movement therapy, while an ongoing six-week exercise group was used as a control. Although the results for mild depressive symptoms are not statistically conclusive, improvements in movement initiation are noted during the dance/movement therapy sessions.

204 Wise, S. K. (1981). Integrating the use of music in movement therapy for patients with spinal cord injuries. *American Journal of Dance Therapy*, *4*(1), 42-51.

The author suggests that music improvisation and imagery be used within dance/movement therapy when working with patients with paralysis. Issues arising from spinal cord injuries include dependency, the mourning process, and the ability to adapt to psychosocial changes. Case examples are given demonstrating music as means to facilitate the expression of emotions when paralysis limits authentic movement.

CHAPTER 13
SUBSTANCE ABUSE

205 Fisher, B. (1990). Dance/movement therapy: It's use in a 28-day substance abuse program. <u>The Arts in Psychotherapy</u>, <u>17</u>(4), 325-331.

The author recommends the use of dance/movement therapy as a support for AA (Alcoholics Anonymous) or other 12 step programs. Focus is placed on dance/movement therapy as an effective aid in facilitating the first step in which abusers accept powerlessness over the substance and admit that their lives are unmanageable. Dance/movement therapy creates movement toward this goal by expanding modes of expressions, creating a nurturing environment for change, supporting a state of receptiveness, encouraging spontaneity, exploring options and decreasing isolation. The author uses a developmental framework as well as case examples to clarify her recommendation.

Harris, J. (Ed.). (1978). Conference proceedings. <u>American Journal of Dance Therapy</u>, <u>2</u>(2), 1-47.

+125

206 Milliken, R. (1990). Dance/movement therapy with the substance abuser. <u>The Arts in Psychotherapy</u>, <u>17</u>(4), 309-317.

The author suggests dance/movement therapy as an effective approach to addressing the issues of substance abusers. Issues presented by the author include lack of body awareness, low self-esteem, resistance and denial. Article defines substance abuse and describes the population in terms of affect, defenses, isolation and movement characteristics. A model for a short-term inpatient program is presented. Group themes (e.g., fear, control and dependency) and the therapist's potential countertransference responses to these surfacing issues are explored.

207   Potocek, J. & Wilder, V. N. (1989). Art/movement psychotherapy in the treatment of the chemically dependent patient. <u>The Arts in Psychotherapy</u>, <u>16</u>(2), 99-103.

                 The use of art and movement therapy as treatment modalities are explored in an Alcoholics Anonymous based 28-day inpatient program. Interventions in movement and art are offered while working with the first four steps of AA on issues of powerlessness, external support, motivation, clarity of purpose, commitment and recognition of strengths and weaknesses in the self and others.

208   Reiland, J. D. (1990). A preliminary study of dance/movement therapy with field dependent alcoholic women. <u>The Arts in Psychotherapy</u>, <u>17</u>(4), 349-354.

                 Two hypotheses are presented suggesting that field dependent alcoholic women will not have articulated body concepts, and that dance/movement therapy will increase articulation and detail in these women's perception of themselves, their bodies and the environment. Subjects were women in a short-term inpatient alcoholic unit of a private psychiatric hospital. Subjects received six one-hour dance/movement therapy sessions. The results of this preliminary study support the hypothesis.

CHAPTER 14
TRAUMATIC BRAIN INJURY

209 Berrol, C. (1990). Dance/movement therapy in head injured rehabilitation. Brain Injury, 4(3), 257-265.

The author uses dance/movement therapy from a neurophysiological perspective in the treatment of the head injured. Maintaining that the psyche and soma are interdependent, the author presents an in-depth case illustration of a client who sustained severe brain damage. A case example includes an emotional and physical evaluation of the client, as well as physical, cognitive and emotional goals for treatment. Therapeutic interventions include the establishment of a secure environment, proprioceptive exercises, the use of space and rhythm, and explorations using eye focus. The author concludes with a follow-up of the client two years post-treatment, and a discussion and summary exploring dance/movement therapy from a neurophysiological perspective for persons with severe brain damage.

210 Berrol, C. F. & Katz, S. S. (1985). Dance/movement therapy in the rehabilitation of individuals surviving severe head injuries. American Journal Dance Therapy, 8, 46-66.

Dance/movement therapy is described in terms of working with patients with severe head injuries. The article provides background information on the consequences of severe head trauma including disorientation, anger, hostility, frustration, confusion and fear. The authors create a framework for dance/movement therapy with this population. Specific foci of therapeutic work are suggested (e.g., body image, motor planning, movement dynamics, spatial organization, feelings and emotions). Examples of individual and group therapy support the use of dance/movement therapy as rehabilitative.

Weisbrod, J. (1972). Shaping body image through movement therapy. Music Educators Journal, 58(8), 66-69.

+155

APPENDIX A

ADDITIONAL CITATIONS

*These articles can also be found in:

Chaiklin, H. (Ed). (1975). <u>Marian Chace: Her Papers</u>. Columbia, MD: American Dance Therapy Association.

American Dance Therapy Association. (1989). <u>A collection of early writings: Toward a body of knowledge</u>. Volume I. Columbia, MD: American Dance Therapy Association.

American Dance Therapy Association. (1988). Moving in health. Monograph No. 4 and Selected Presentations of <u>the 22nd Annual Conference of the American Dance Therapy Association</u>. Columbia, MD: American Dance Therapy Association.

American Dance Therapy Association. (1989). Moving into a new decade: Dance/movement therapy in the 90's. <u>Monograph No. 6 and Conference Abstracts of the 24th Annual Conference and 2nd International Conferences of the American Dance Therapy Association</u>. Columbia, MD: American Dance Therapy Association.

Bernstein, P. L. (1972). <u>Theory and methods in dance/movement therapy</u>. Dubuque, IA: Kendall/Hunt.

Campbell, D. (1934). Psychology and the modern dance. <u>Dance Observer</u>, <u>73</u>, 76-77.

*Chace, M. (1954). Common principles in music therapy. <u>Music Therapy</u>, <u>4</u>, 87-90.

*Chace, M. (1958). Dance in growth or treatment settings. <u>Music Therapy</u>, <u>8</u>, 119-122.

*Chace, M. (1951). Dance therapy at St. Elizabeths Hospital. <u>The Psychiatric Aide</u>, <u>8</u>(9), 3-4.

*Chace, M. (1958). Development of group interaction through dance. In J. H. Masserman and J. L. Moreno (Eds.), <u>Progress in Psychotherapy-Technique of Psychiatry: Vol. 3</u>. (pp.149-153). New York: Grune and Stratton.

*Chace, M. (1955). Hotel St. Elizabeths: a unique experiment in therapy. <u>Americas</u>, <u>7</u>, 36.

Chace, M. (1961). Leadership in dance sessions within an institutional setting. *Yearbook of Brooklyn College Association for Health and Physical Education, 2*, 20-23, 27-28.

*Chace, M. (1958). Measurable and intangible aspects of dance sessions. In E. T. Gaston (Ed.), *Music therapy 1957: Seventh book of proceedings of the national association for music therapy, Inc.* (pp. 264-275). Lawrence, KS: National Association of Music Therapy, Inc.

*Chace, M. (1967, November). Music in dance therapy. *Music Journal*, 25-26.

*Chace, M. (1952). Physiological aspects. *Music Therapy, 2*, 63-67.

*Chace, M. (1954). Report of group project, St. Elizabeths Hospital. *Music Therapy, 4*, 187-190.

*Chace, M. (1945). Rhythm in movement as used in St. Elizabeths Hospital. In J. L. Moreno (Ed.), *Group psychotherapy, a symposium* (pp. 243-245). New York: Beacon House.

*Chace, M. (1958). Stimulation of creative forms in patient production. *Bulletin of the National Association for Music Therapy, 7*, 9-10.

*Chace, M. (1964, June). The power of movement with others. *Dance Magazine, 38*, 42-45, 68-69.

*Chace, M. (1960). The role of the psychiatric nurse in dance sessions. *SNANYS Newsletter, 8*(6), 8-9.

*Chace, M. (1962). The structuring of dance sessions for varying needs of patients. *Music Therapy, 12*, 63-68.

*Chace, M. (1953). Techniques for the use of dance as a group therapy. *Music Therapy, 3*, 62-67.

*Chace, M. & Bunney, J. (1962). Some observations on the psychodrama sessions at Chestnut Lodge. *Eighth Annual Chestnut Lodge Symposium*, 19-31.

*Chace, M. & Johnson, W. R. (1961). Our real lives are lived in movement. *Journal of Health, Physical Education and Recreation, 32*, 3-9.

Chujoy, A. (Ed.). (1949). *Dance as therapy: Dance encyclopedia*. New York: Barnes and Company.

Cole, I. L. & Thomas, D. (Eds.). (1981). Research as a creative process: Implications for dance therapy theory and practice. *Compendium of Presenter's Abstracts, 16th Annual Conference of the American Dance Therapy Association*. Columbia, MD: American Dance Therapy Association.

Committee on Research in Dance. (1972). Dance therapy bibliography. *Cord News, 4*(2).

Davis, M. & Skupien, J. (Eds.). (1981). *The nonverbal communication literature 1971-80: Annotated bibliography of the behavioral study of body movement*. New York: Arno Press.

Dosamantes-Alperson, E. (1979). Bodily-experiencing and hypnogogic imagery in experiential movement therapy. *Bulletin of the American Association for the Study of Mental Imagery, 2*(1), 1-3.

Dulicai, D. (1973). Movement analysis as a diagnostic evaluation with intensive care patients. *Albert Einstein Medical Journal, 1*(1), 22-27.

Dulicai, D. (?). Movement analysis in understanding a family system. *Devereaux Papers, 3*(1). 120-133.

Feher, M. (1949, May). The dancer's anatomy: Dance therapy for disabled dancers. *Dance Magazine*, pp. 28-29, 32.

Genther, S. (1954). A place to begin. *Impulse*, 19-22.

Greenburg, T. R. & Berlin, A. L. (1980). *Move! Dance is therapy*. Berkeley, CA: Center Press.

Helm, J. & Gill, K. (1974). An essential resource for aging. *Dance Research Journal of Committee on Research in Dance, 7*(1), 1-7.

Henrick, R. (Ed.). (1980). <u>Psychotherapy handbook</u>. New York: New American Library.

Kavaler, S. (1974). Dance therapy with retarded children. <u>International Mental Health Newsletter</u>, <u>16</u>(1), 9-11.

Kelly, M. (1982, May). The movement toward dance therapy. <u>Minneapolis - St. Paul Magazine</u>, <u>10</u>, 69.

Levine, F. (1980). Dance therapy: Focus on process. <u>Compendium of Presenters Abstracts, 15th Annual Conference of the American Dance Therapy Association</u>. Columbia, MD: American Dance Therapy Association.

Melville, T. R. (1987). Dancing the blues away: Dance and dance therapy. <u>Dance Theater Journal</u>, <u>5</u>(2), 25.

Minar, V., et.al. (1978). <u>Expressive therapies: The arts and the exceptional child. An annotated bibliography</u>. Washington, DC: Department of Health, Education and Welfare.

Mossman, M. & Silberman, L. (1976). Movement - the joyous language: Dance therapy for children. <u>Children's House Magazine</u>, <u>8</u>(5), 11-16.

National Library of Medicine (U.S.). (Ed.). (1970). <u>The arts in therapy: Including art, literature, poetry, drama, music, and dance as used as therapy, rehabilitation, or analgesia, January 1968 through September 1970</u>. Bethesda, MD: National Institute of Health.

Ohwaki, S. (1976). An assessment of dance therapy to improve retarded adults' body image. <u>Perceptual and Motor Skills</u>, <u>43</u>(3), 1122.

Penfield, K. (1986). The growth of dance therapy in Europe. <u>Ballet International</u>, <u>9</u>(4), 10-11.

Perlmutter, R. (1974). Dance me a cloud. <u>Children's House Magazine</u>, <u>6</u>(6), 15-19.

Robbins, A. (Ed.). (1980). <u>Crossroads in expressive arts therapy</u>. New York: Science House.

Sandel, S. L. (1980). Dance therapy in the psychiatric hospital. *National Association of Private Psychiatric Hospitals Journal*, 11(2), 20-26.

Schmais, C. & Orleans, F. (1978). *Dance therapy research: Seven pilot studies*. New York: Hunter College.

Shorr, J. E., et.al. (Eds.). (1980). *Imagery: It's many dimensions and applications*. New York: Plenum Press.

Stern, E. (1959). Dance of release. *Coronet Magazine*, 45, 96-100.

Vislocky, D. (1970). *American dance therapy association bibliography*. Columbia, MD: American Dance Therapy Association.

Weiner, C. (1973). *Dance/movement therapy bibliography*. New York: Gowanda State Hospital.